EASY PEASY HEALTHY EATING

The Busy Parents' Guide to Helping Picky Eaters Love Vegetables

Julie Schooler

DISCLAIMER

This healthy eating guide is designed to give parents and caregivers some useful tips and ideas. It does not replace expert advice from medical or behavioral specialists. It is recommended that you seek advice from qualified practitioners if you are concerned in any way.

This book is dedicated to my sister, Karen, who has bewitched all three of her children into eating Brussels sprouts.

CONTENTS

READER GIFT: THE HAPPY20

For all you wonderful, busy parents, I created

THE HAPPY20
20 Free Ways to Boost Happiness in 20 Seconds or Less

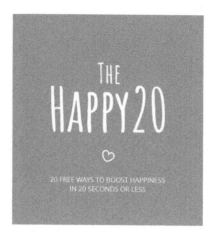

A PDF gift for you with quick ideas to improve mood and add a little sparkle to your day.

Head to **JulieSchooler.com/gift** and grab your copy today.

1

BRING HEALTHY BACK

> 66 *'It is easier to build strong children than to repair broken men.'* – Frederick Douglass

FIX THE FUSSY

Does your child hate eating vegetables? Are mealtimes a constant struggle to get nutritious food into your family? Do you want your kids to effortlessly eat healthy food every day but instead find yourself begging, bribing or bellowing just to get vegetables past their lips?

This book is filled with the best strategies plus fun, easy and practical tips to get your fussy child, and the whole family, to eat lots more vegetables every day—and love it.

It also cuts through the confusion around healthy eating, provides compelling reasons why upping your vegetable intake is important and tell you how to avoid picky eating and food battles.

You won't need to spend hours searching for information all over the Internet, and by the end you will have a clear direction and won't be confused by all the conflicting advice. There is no need to repeat common mistakes made by other parents.

WHY THIS BOOK WAS WRITTEN

I am not a nutritionist or dietician, and I don't have a medical background. My family will definitely agree that I am no gourmet chef. I am simply a mother of two children. My wish is that they grow up as healthy as possible.

After too many dinnertime struggles and rejections when a nutritious meal over which I had slaved was refused, I knew there must be a better way to get my kids to eat healthy every day without the stress.

So I did what I always do: I read. A lot. I read books, newspaper and magazine articles; I searched all over the Internet and even went to seminars on health and wellbeing. I also surveyed dozens of other parents. I then distilled the avalanche of advice into simple and practical tips to get your kids to eat more vegetables and enjoy it.

Why have I done this? Because I had to. Surprisingly, I could not find one short, clear, gimmick-free guide to eating healthier with the focus on vegetables. This is the book I wish I had a few years back. Luckily, it is not too late. I have already started using the strategies in this book to create healthy changes for my little family.

BENEFITS

Just think how great it will be when your little one is eating vegetables every day without a struggle. There are benefits in so many areas:

- As a parent – you can pat yourself on the back as your child develops lifelong healthy eating habits.
- Your children – they are healthy and happy (what more could you possibly want?)
- Environment – eating more vegetables is good for the planet.
- Time – more time to spend with your family doing fun things and not fighting over mealtimes.
- Money – more cold hard cash available as you are not throwing away uneaten food or spending it on takeaways.

Other parents are happy to recommend this one, easy-to-read, concise guide. Most say it is refreshing that there are no mandatory instructions of what must or must not be done.

The book lays out dozens of tips from which any family can select, along with the reasons why they are good ideas.

Parents are excited that there is finally a short book that gives them options for increasing their family's vegetable intake in a stress-free way.

My Promise to You

My promise is that if you use even a couple of the tips in this book, your children will eat more vegetables, mealtimes will be happier, and you will give your children the best gift of all—a longer, healthier life.

If we can't have a bit of fun and enjoyment during a time when, yet again, you are tearing your hair out just to get your youngster to eat one pea, then it is a sad life indeed. So my next promise to you is that not only will this be easy, but you will also have a bit of a laugh along the way.

WHAT HAVE YOU GOT TO LOSE?

Let's face it, how much do you really want to read on this subject? All you need to know has been chunked down into quick, straightforward chapters.

Do not prepare dinner tonight without reading this book first. Do it right from now on and blast into a healthy future today.

WHEN NOT TO READ THIS BOOK

> *'There are two types of people; those who eat kale and those who should.'* - Bo Muller-Moore

A KALE TALE

This book starts with a tale about kale.

Yes, kale. A bitter, leafy green superfood with tons of goodness... *but* only if it is actually ingested by a human being. You cannot attain all the nutrients and antioxidants and unicorn magical sprinkles from kale if it is not actually placed into the mouth, chewed, swallowed and digested.

So you probably think I had set myself an insurmountable challenge when, a few months ago, I decided to introduce this vegetable to my three-year-old. However, I remembered a simple recipe, pulled it out, adjusted it a bit and created 'Kale Chips', which I promptly served up to Master Three.

The result—a little voice requesting, most politely: "More kale chips, please".

That was said after months and months of dinnertime battles, total food refusal and inexplicable fussiness (loves carrots one day, rejects them the next). It was uttered just when all the worry, guilt, stress and frustration of trying to feed my family healthy food every day was starting to peak. It happened when I had little energy, time and inspiration to keep trying much longer. However, that appeal from my beautiful son suddenly made all my efforts worthwhile.

It also started me thinking, there has to be a better way. I decided I must be onto something. And so this book began. I wanted to research and collate the most effective, yet effortless methods to get kids to eat healthier.

The initial quest took me straight to vegetables.

WHY ONLY VEGETABLES?

Eating vegetables is:

- universally recognized as the most crucial part of a healthy and nutritious lifestyle, and
- almost impossible to actually get our children to do easily and consistently.

This core conflict is the cause of misery and despair for parents everywhere. It is one thing to know what our children should eat and quite another to get them to actually eat it. Hence why vegetables are the focus of this book.

Even with the focus on vegetables, there are still a number of questions, such as how much should be served, which vegetables are best, and should you worry if it is organic or not? All this will be discussed soon.

WHAT THIS BOOK IS NOT ABOUT

I do not want to waste your time, so read through this list to decide if this is the book for you.

This book is a no-nonsense overview of research findings and parental wisdom around vegetables translated into practical recommendations for parents of kids aged about two to twelve. It is NOT for babies who can only eat pureed or mushy food. However, it may still be helpful with the odd stubborn teenager.

It is packed with useful facts, clever tips, inspiring ideas and quite a few tasty recipes, but it is NOT a cookbook.

It discusses lots of ways of including vegetables into meals, but it is NOT vegan or vegetarian as such. Although being paleo or pescatarian or gluten-free are trendy concepts these days, this book does not advocate any particular diet. The word 'diet' has so many confusing and possibly negative associations that it will rarely be used.

The book will help with typical fussy kids, which can include almost no vegetable eating at all, but it is NOT for severely picky eaters who may have a medical problem or anyone who requires a special diet due to intolerances or allergies. If you are concerned that your child may have a medical or behavioral issue that prevents her from eating well, then seek professional help. In saying that, most families will benefit from the tips to up their vegetable intake in here.

The main focus of this book is on helping kids to eat and love vegetables, so if your child is already great at this, then this book may NOT be for you. However, if Junior instead has a problem with fruit or meat or a specific food, then you can still use most of the strategies.

This book does not list every vitamin and mineral lurking in our greens, nor supply definitions of what a carbohydrate or protein is. It is NOT a dusty textbook full of dull science. Instead it takes the best recommendations from studies and parents, combined with some interesting facts about vegetables to give a short, practical and easy-to-read guide for busy parents.

The astute amongst you may have realized this already, but this book is NOT just for your children. Parents, the extended family and your entire community could benefit from the strategies contained in here.

Know that this book is NOT stopping you or your family from eating fast food, junk food, treat food or whatever you call it. Feel free to eat it occasionally, and absolutely relish it when you do. But you may find that when you start to eat healthier, you will feel satisfied and naturally will not crave those sorts of foods as much.

HOUSEKEEPING

Vegetables are eaten as part of balanced and healthy diet. This means that everyone should also eat correct portions of protein (meat, fish, milk, eggs, legumes, etc.), carbohydrates (potato, pasta, rice, bread, etc.) and (good) fats (olive oil, oily fish, nuts), plus of course some fruit.

The trouble is that many people have a way higher proportion of carbohydrates and fat and a way lower proportion of vegetables, and this is what this book seeks to redress.

When discussing which vegetables to eat, the focus here is on non-starchy vegetables which this book singles out as potato (there are others, but potato is the main one). Think of potato as a carbohydrate, not a vegetable.

This book talks about vegetables in the conventional sense, so some vegetables that are technically fruits, such as tomatoes and avocados, are referred to as vegetables.

This book is for parents and caregivers of children aged between two and twelve years old. Your child will be addressed in a number of different ways including:

- child
- kid
- youngster
- little one
- young one
- Junior
- tiny human

It also means that sometimes I refer to your child as 'he' and sometimes as 'she'. The use of he or she has been alternated throughout the book. If a section, story or paragraph refers to 'he' and your child is a 'she,' then change the pronoun in your head (and vice versa).

Throughout the book are scattered some Mama and Daddy stories and tips. Look for these little gems in *italics*. They are often helpful, sometimes hilarious and always honest tales from those in the trenches.

Now we have weeded out who this book is NOT for, let's tackle the problems that you may have.

3

EATING AND MEALTIME TROUBLE

> *'I do not like green eggs and ham! I do not like them Sam-I-am.'* – Dr. Seuss

VEGETABLE ISSUES

Do any, or perhaps ALL, of the following problems sound familiar?

Is there one or more fussy eater in your house? Does your picky little one eat almost no vegetables at all, or does he consume only a small array of favorite vegetables (often prepared or cooked in a certain way)?

Is dinner a battlefield, full of stress and conflict? Do you find yourself pleading, nagging, or even worse, yelling at your kids?

Do you dread trying to quickly prepare something

each night that the family will all be happy about, or at least eat, before everyone rushes off to the next thing?

Are you upset that your lovingly prepared, nutritious meal has been rejected once again? Are you sick of being a cheerleader for healthy food that no one eats?

Do you resort to bribing the kids with sweet treats and dessert just to get some greens into them, but then feel guilty afterwards?

Are you confused with the avalanche of contradictory information and not sure what is 'right' anymore? Does the advice seem hard to stick to or too time consuming when you are not sure if the results are even worth it?

Do you always worry that your little one has not eaten enough and that she will get hungry-angry or 'hangry' later? Or do you worry that if she doesn't eat much she will be malnourished or not have all of the nutrients she needs to function well?

Is it frustrating to find that just because your kids like the taste of a vegetable it does not mean they will eat it? Do they eat something one day only to reject it the next day (or week or month)?

Do you find yourself hiding vegetables in favorite foods more and more, or shoveling food in while your kid watches TV, just so that he eats something nutritious without the fight? Do you worry that he may never recognize a carrot or wonder if this no-conflict stance is sending the right message?

Mama Story - All of my four kids have likes and dislikes. One of them went through a stage where she would not eat anything yellow. - Nora

So why is food in general, and eating vegetables in particular, so rife with problems? Why do so many parents despair over their kids' picky habits? Why do so many adults have poor relationships with food that often lead to health and weight issues?

Actually, it is not surprising that this is the case. Food, eating, feeding and mealtimes are connected to power issues, high emotion and wonky ingrained belief systems. When these three factors are taken into account, it is a wonder that anyone has a great relationship with food at all. The first two are tackled below, and as beliefs can play an enormous part in these issues, they have the next chapter all to themselves.

FOOD AND POWER

A very young child doesn't have complete control over much in her day-to-day life, but she can control what goes in her mouth, chews and swallows. And once she works this out—and it's often very early on—good luck getting her to eat anything she has decided against. We can choose the healthiest meal, put it on her plate and sometimes even get it into her mouth, but if she decides that's as far as it goes, then game over.

Our tiny humans are meant to progressively become more independent, but when it shines through at mealtimes, eating and feeding can easily fall into a power struggle. The phrase 'will of steel' comes to mind, even with an otherwise placid and compliant child.

If you decide to participate in the power struggle, you are often rewarding the less-than-desirable behavior—which can range from a calm food refusal right through to spitting and throwing—with your attention. This is not an optimal outcome when all you want is for her is to eat a couple of beans. Your child has not only successfully asserted who is the boss in this particular arena, but has managed to wind you up in the process.

But don't despair, help is at hand. There are lots of great techniques for frustrated parents in the strategies outlined in this book. This includes ideas that may sound like the opposite of what you would think, like allowing your kids to make some decisions on eating for themselves, giving them more control in their lives, and saying YES more often.

FOOD AND EMOTIONS

You lovingly prepare a meal for your child and it is thunderously rejected. First, you start to fear for your tiny human. When he refuses to do the most basic yet necessary act of eating, it can be really frightening. You worry that he will starve, be malnourished, or have a 'hangry' tantrum due to lack of food. You know you need to support his growth and development, and it stresses you out when he flat out refuses the nutritious 'fuel' that you supply. On top of that, making a nutritious meal that gets refused can create feelings of sadness, rejection, frustration and distress for the chef.

I am not going to tell you to take the emotion out of it; how can you? Feeding your child is packed with feelings because it relates to the core of being a parent—nurturing, responsibility and ultimately love. You are trying to feed your young one vegetables because you LOVE him or her.

FOOD IS LOVE.

Feel your emotions, let them come and then release them. This is one day of many, many days of being a parent, and tomorrow you will likely feel differently. It is easy to tell people to relax and it's very hard to do, but give yourself a break: you are a wonderful parent.

And please know this—there are many reasons why a child rejects food, and it is extremely unlikely that your child means it as a rejection of you or your love. For instance, he could simply not be hungry. Maybe he has snacked too much during the day, or he could be unwell or not like the smell or texture of the food. As noted above, this could be a power play or an angry response about something. Or he may just be busy playing and does not want to leave what he is doing.

If all this does not lift your spirits, then read on for some superb tips that will stop the refusal of vegetables and the feelings of rejection that go with it. There is nothing better than the feeling you get when you create a nutritious meal and your whole family demolishes it and asks for more.

Before we get started on the strategies, it is important to look at your beliefs and behaviors around food.

4

BELIEFS

'*The trouble with eating Italian is that five or six days later, you're hungry again.*' – George Miller

CHECK YOUR BELIEF SYSTEM

All of us carry a bunch of beliefs about food, eating and mealtimes from our childhoods into our parenthoods. Some of these are great habits, and some of these may subconsciously create issues.

This chapter spells out some common beliefs and questions whether they are still serving you and your family today.

THE PICKY EATER

Maybe you were called a picky or fussy eater growing up. Some of you may now enjoy a wide variety of foods and some of you not so much. There are two beliefs around picky eaters that may or may not be true. But truth does not matter. What is important is whether they still work for you.

First—do you believe that picky eaters will 'grow out of it'? This is possibly a good belief to cling to, but if your child refuses to entertain the notion of trying different foods, especially vegetables, this belief can allow you to passively ignore the problem. Sure, some kids may 'get over it' as they get older, but maybe they won't. Plus, isn't it good to try and encourage variety when they are young? Don't worry about whether it is possible—there are plenty of strategies in here that you can try—the main thing is to decide whether this belief is helping your current situation and if you want to change it.

Second—labels stick. Once your child hears that she is a picky eater, she absorbs the label and decides that it is part of who she is. Once a label is placed, it is much harder to shift her perspective and behavior. Labeling a fussy eater makes the situation sound more permanent than it really is. Instead, create a temporary observation, for example, "Jessie does not like beans right now, but we are working on it".

BLAND FOOD

There seems to be a culturally accepted belief in the USA, Canada, UK, Australia, New Zealand and perhaps a few other countries, that children only like bland food. Please throw this thought out of your head; it is complete garbage.

Why wouldn't kids like bright colors when they enjoy them with toys and games? Why wouldn't they enjoy tasting different vegetables when pre-packaged foods are often stronger in flavor than naturally grown ones?

Even if you thought it was 'true', it does nothing to help you. It discourages you from getting your kids to try new foods and can often lead to becoming a 'short order cook', making different meals for the kids and the adults in the household. It almost certainly means fewer vegetables will be offered, as the richly colored ones would not be considered bland enough.

Why not take a positive approach and assume that kids can actually enjoy eating a wide variety of foods—that they could like the subtle flavor of broccoli? What have you got to lose? In France, they truly believe that children inherently like the rich world of flavors in most foods. Let your child have the opportunity to give each food a chance.

THE CLEAN PLATE CLUB

Like many people growing up, we were encouraged to 'clean our plates'. One of the clearest memories I have is of my parents stating that they would package up my leftovers and "send them to the starving children in Ethiopia". Sometimes I was cajoled with "just one last mouthful" and sometimes was bribed with dessert. Let me state up front, my parents are wonderful people and were doing the best job they could to get us to eat healthy. Most of the time we scraped our plates clean.

But no matter what they said or did, it did not make me want to eat pumpkin, and in all honestly, I still have a hang-up about that vegetable today. So even though they wanted me to finish all my food, if I dug my toes in about something I especially didn't like, then I would not eat it no matter what.

Think about it—how many foods that you were force-fed during your childhood do you willingly eat now? Force-feeding in any way never ever EVER works. It can often lead to eating LESS as your offspring asserts some independence and control.

Just as bad, The Clean Plate Club can lead to eating MORE. Studies have shown that if you double the amount of food put on their plates, many people will eat 25% more regardless of how hungry they are. One of the researchers who showed this was Brian Wansink. In his book *Mindless Eating*, he demonstrates that children who were required to clean their plates not only ate more than necessary but then went on to eat TWICE as much dessert.

This mentality can stop a child from independently working out when he feels full, which is an essential element to a lifelong great relationship with food. We are born with this natural ability, and it is hard to get back if we start to lose it. Another downside is that 'clean your plate' could even teach kids to lie about still being hungry in order to get to the cake, and then they may start to learn to lie to themselves.

The Clean Plate Club can also get you to start to think of large helpings as normal. Children are growing up today without knowing what a healthy serving size is. Our parents and grandparents may have grown up with scarcity and smaller plates, but for most of us there is an abundance of any food we want.

This is especially frightening when you note the following:

- The average plate size has expanded 36% since 1960.
- New editions of cookbooks with the same recipe for cookies state that it makes 16 cookies when it used to state that it made 30.
- Dishwashers have wider racks and cars have bigger drink holders.
- A typical muffin in the United States is THREE times greater than the USDA recommendation for how big a muffin should be.
- Police are ordering bigger handcuffs as even criminals are getting fatter!

If these facts do not scare you (and I for one find overweight criminals a worry), then as a final note on this subject, understand that finishing your plate is simply a cultural norm. In Thailand it is actually considered rude to clear your plate or to finish all the food on the table. It implies that the host has not provided enough food for her guests. In Thailand it is considered an honor to have leftovers.

WASTE

But, you say, if they don't eat it, it will go to waste. If there is one area you need to change your perception on, then it is so-called 'wasted' food. It is not a major waste of food if your young child does not eat the two stalks of broccoli on her plate.

Over a BILLION tons of food produced for human consumption gets lost or wasted every year. A billion! Your child's waste is not going to significantly impact on that number.

If a billion tons of waste horrifies you, then do something about it in your own small way. Create or buy a worm farm. Have a compost bin in your backyard that can then be used on your vegetable garden (more on growing a garden later). Raise chickens and give leftovers to them, or feed them to the dog later. Or simply eat it yourself—package any leftovers up for lunch the next day.

Besides, it is actually a waste if you overeat, too, because it will come out as waste if your body does not need the excess food.

Mama Tip - I gave Adam raw carrots about a million times and finally he decided he could bear to eat them. Recently he has had the odd mouthful of salad. Repetition and expecting waste. We got chickens because of the amount of food waste from the kids, although interestingly our chickens don't eat vegetables either. – Terri

INFORMATION OVERLOAD

Every day we are bombarded with opinions, advice, guidelines, well-meaning wisdom, and all it does is leave us overwhelmed, confused and uncertain. Not only that, but there are a multitude of food products to choose from. Step into an average supermarket and you are faced with nearly 50,000 items on offer. Yes 50,000! How are we supposed to determine what is healthy? Who has the time to read all those labels?

Up to 75% of children aged two to eight are not consuming recommended servings of vegetables. Over a third of toddlers may not eat any vegetables at all on a given day. In 2010, over 40 million children under five were overweight and the latest figures estimate at least 20% of all children in the world are overweight or obese.

There is something very wrong with a world in which we can have children dying of starvation and an increasing child obesity epidemic. Some kids are both malnourished AND obese at the same time!

I am interested in my health, my children's health, my nation's health, the health of the entire world, but on some days it seems too much. Prepping for a zombie apocalypse seems easier than this!

So let's strip it back to basics. Keep it simple. Start with vegetables.

Vegetables.

That is it.

'But,' you say, 'I don't know which vegetables are best or how much I should be serving up in the first place'. Let's have a detour and look at some of the best types of vegetables plus recommended portion sizes before we get to some of the amazing benefits of eating them.

5

VEGETABLE Q&A

66 'Eat food. Not too much. Mostly plants.' –
Michael Pollan

What are the 'Best' Vegetables to Eat?

You know what I am going to say, don't you?

ALL OF THEM.

Start somewhere. It doesn't matter what you start with.

Just eat more vegetables.

Specifically, most of this book excludes starchy vegetables, and in this case the main item in this category is potatoes. Don't get me wrong, potatoes are great, I just don't think we need to encourage our kids to eat them. It is all the other vegetables with which they take issue.

As a rule of thumb, the more brightly or deeply colored the vegetable is, the more nutritional value it has. If you want to hone in the best of the best, then these are the three main suggestions:

- Cruciferous family—superfoods that actively fight cancer—includes broccoli, cabbage, cauliflower and everybody's favorite, Brussels sprouts.
- Dark leafy green vegetables—includes kale, spinach, broccoli, chard (silverbeet), etc.
- Bright orange and red vegetables—includes carrots, tomato, pumpkin, pepper (capsicum), squash, beets, etc.

Sometimes spinach and pumpkin are a hard-sell to kids, so if you want to give yourself more chance of winning the vegetable battle, then the top five vegetables for nutrition AND kid friendliness are red pepper, baby carrots, broccoli, tomatoes and snap peas. Also popular with the kids but slightly less nutritious are green beans, peas, corn, cucumber and lettuce.

Don't get too hung up about this. It is the daily routine of eating vegetables—ANY vegetables—that is most important.

DO I NEED TO FEED MY CHILDREN ORGANIC?

You know what I am going to say, don't you?

NO.

It is very difficult to know whether what you are buying is truly organic in the first place. Plus, it has not been proven that organic vegetables significantly improve health outcomes compared with non-organic. There is also less of a selection of organic vegetables available, and they are often more expensive. What this adds up to is that people who try to eat organic end up eating FEWER vegetables than people who don't.

You are already doing enough by trying to up your family's vegetable intake. Get that sorted first, and then if the organic thing is still playing on your mind, see what you can do to introduce more organically grown vegetables into your meals. Perhaps start with fruit and vegetables you eat with the skin on, like apples. Or grow your own vegetable garden, which is discussed later in the book.

In the meantime, wash with water before preparing and eating. If you are particularly concerned about pesticide residue, then wash with three parts water to one part vinegar. This is best done with a bunch of vegetables in your kitchen sink. Then rinse with fresh water and pat dry before preparing or storing.

What are the Recommended Serving or Portion Sizes for Vegetables?

You know what I am going to say, don't you?

Actually, you probably don't.

Like most information out there, there is a wealth of confusing and conflicting suggestions when it comes to vegetables and how much we should eat. Take a look at these headlines, both from *The Telegraph* newspaper in the UK, and spaced only a few months apart:

> *'Healthy diet means 10 portions of fruit and vegetables per day, not five' (31 March 2014)*

'A five a day diet of fruit and vegetables is best – more is pointless, study finds' (30 July 2014)

This would be hilarious if it wasn't such a life and death issue. So where do we start? Please note that it is IMPOSSIBLE to know how much your own children need to eat over a daily, weekly, monthly or yearly basis. Your job is to serve up nutritious food, and their job is to work out how much of it they eat. This 'Division of Responsibility', promoted by Ellyn Satter, will be detailed in the 'Accept and Allow' chapter.

Daily guidelines are specified below, but it is important to look at the big picture. Day to day, children can vary in their want and need for food. They can eat everything in sight one day and eat like a bird the next. This is perfectly normal. It is over a week or a month that they should consume the nutrition they need.

> *Mama Tip – I wish parents would understand the fact that you need to look at a whole week to get a true picture on nutrition. Never look at a single day, unless it's a good day - then congratulate yourself! – Annabelle.*

We have all heard of the '5+ A Day' recommendation, but what does it actually mean? This is the directive from the World Health Organization (WHO) and it means five portions of fruit and vegetables per day.

Of this, at least three portions should be vegetables. A portion size is about a handful, and for children, it is the size of their hand. On top of this, WHO really loves dark green vegetables and orange fruit or vegetables and advises us to incorporate these into the 5+ A Day.

So WHO recommends a minimum consumption of three handfuls of vegetables per day. A handful for a very little person is one small carrot, two large spears of broccoli or three beans or cherry tomatoes. Three handfuls roughly translates to one cup of vegetables per day for under fives and one and a half to two cups for five-to-twelve-year-olds.

Depending on where you are currently, this could seem like an unattainable goal, or not that much at all. However, remember this is an absolute minimum requirement. When it comes to vegetables (despite the headlines above), the more the better.

Nutritional expert and health guru Dr. Libby Weaver states:

> *"Most people can very safely and beneficially **double** the amount of vegetables they currently eat".*

This translates to three to eight servings (i.e. large handfuls) of different seasonal vegetables as part of meals and snacks throughout the day. Or another way to think about it is for lunch and dinner, half the plate should be non-starchy vegetables.

In summary – aim for an intake of **one to two cups of vegetables per day** for your tiny human. This can be split between meals (more on this later).

> *Mama Story – I find I have two grazers and two who eat three good meals a day. When you look at it they are all eating around the same amount – Nora.*

Now that we know what sorts of vegetables to eat, and how much, let's get to WHY we should eat them in the first place. Don't worry, this is not tedious science, but interesting tidbits you can tell your kids.

6

BENEFITS OF VEGETABLES

> 'Let your food be thy medicine, and medicine be thy food.' - Hippocrates

So Many Benefits

Before we get to the amazing health benefits of vegetables it is worth noting that by focusing on what we can do—eat more vegetables—we stop obsessing about what to avoid and instead celebrate healthy deliciousness.

This in itself is an awesome benefit. We are focusing on MORE, not less—MORE real food.

Everyone knows and agrees that eating lots of vegetables is good for you. It is so well known it has become a cliché in our society. But we are at least on the same page that vegetables are good for you, right?

Right?

Headline from a Guardian newspaper article from 2002:

'Research links cancer to fruit and vegetables'

Well, maybe not every single one of us. Excluding that one article (which was based on a single, non-replicated study) the health benefits of vegetables are hard to ignore.

The problem is that we tend to present these to our kids as a lecture that seems preachy, dull and not that relevant. One study shows that when lectured about the merits of eating vegetables, kids assumed they would taste bad and were even more resistant to them.

We need a 'What's In It For Me' or 'WIIFM' approach.

WIIFM

As parents we need to get past the 'high antioxidants', 'loads of iron' or 'contains all the Vitamin C you need today' arguments and tell our kids how these attributes help their little bodies. Phytochemicals, vitamins, minerals and fiber are all nebulous concepts that are hard to imagine and quantify, so let's skip these middle men and go straight from vegetable to cool result.

Here is a list of WIIFM vegetable facts. The final word on this is to only drop them into conversations sparingly and try to be cool about it. Be. Cool.

VEGETABLES IN GENERAL ARE SLAM DUNK AMAZING

If someone were to tell you that to reduce the risk of cancer, heart disease and diabetes as well as strengthen your eyes, bones, muscles and organs and support your immune system, you had to take a few pills each and every day, you would think it was too good to be true.

But when you eat a just a few portions of vegetables each day, that is exactly what you are doing. Vegetables make you **healthier**.

What else do they do?

Vegetables make you **smarter**—they help with brain function, mental health, alertness and concentration.

Vegetables make you **nicer**—they are slow to digest and prevent blood sugar highs and lows, which reduces tantrums and whining and improves overall mood.

Vegetables make you more **good-looking**—they are full of vitamins, minerals and other goodness that builds clear, glowing skin, sparkling eyes, silky hair and promotes strong nail growth.

Some Vegetables in Particular are Slam Dunk Amazing

Avocado (although technically a fruit) has more potassium than a banana and half the fiber a three-year-old needs each day. It is the only vegetable that contains monounsaturated fat (a 'good' fat). The vitamin E in it actively helps heal cuts, not to mention prevents brittle hair and nails.

Beets (Beetroot) have antioxidants to protect cells, folic acid to grow cells and potassium and nitrate to regulate blood pressure—all this means in kid language is more energy to play ball.

Broccoli and **cauliflower** are two of the main vegetables that are part of the Brassica family. This family of superfoods not only has a ton of vitamin C to heal cuts and calcium for strong, healthy teeth, but also contains cancer-fighting properties.

Butternut, squash and **pumpkin**, especially the ones with the deep orange color, contain tons of beta carotene that improves eyesight. Tell your kids they will be able to see the moon and stars better at night. Also, the high potassium improves heart health, so tell your little ones that it helps them to play outside for longer without getting tired.

Carrots, as everyone knows, are packed with beta carotene, which promotes good eyesight, so Junior can be 'like Superman with X-Ray vision' (just be careful about over-selling these benefits).

Kale is packed with vitamins that include most letters of the alphabet, including A, C and E. It also contains magnesium and calcium, which are critical to helping us relax, so kale may even help our kids to bliss out!

Peas are great for the heart and also for digestion. They keep everything regular and moving – tell your kids that peas help them poop!

Peppers are very high in vitamin C, which fights infections so your child is not miserable with colds and other illnesses.

Spinach not only has a lot of iron so your child can be as strong as Popeye, but folic acid that helps cell growth and lutein for improved vision (also like Superman). One cup gives you the recommended daily serving of calcium for adults.

Sprouts and **zucchini** (courgettes) have fantastic qualities like vitamin C, calcium, magnesium and phosphorus, which lead to clear, glowing skin.

Tomato has so many benefits that it is hard to choose what to promote, but one thing it does is increase the proportion of vitamin C in the blood, which inhibits the levels of stress hormones, hence it eases tension and stress.

THE AMAZING VEGETABLE

When it comes to food, nature gets it right. Eating vegetables means you are eating food that is ALIVE. We are designed to absorb nutrients from living foods and plants. Incorporating more plant foods into our daily lives is the quickest and easiest way to increase our intake of the nutrients our bodies need. Plus eating more real food reduces the frequency of eating packaged and processed foods and all the harmful substances they potentially contain.

It is win-win.

Deep down, we all know that eating plants makes us feel good. If we listen to our body, we can hear it craving for vegetables. We thrive when we eat real, living food.

And if all of this is not enough to convince your kids it's a good idea, then tell them this one last fact: gorillas have a 50% plant-based diet and they have one of the highest muscle masses of any living creature. In other words, EAT PLANTS = POWERFUL AND STRONG. And who doesn't want that?

Daddy Story - We have a mantra: 'vegetables make you

strong'. If the kids think they're finished then sometimes we check their biceps and advise them they need to eat a little more – Rob.

Now that you are excited about eating vegetables, you may be wondering how you can get Junior to eat them. Let's decide on some goals. Yes goals for eating vegetables. Read on.

7

GOALS

 'Never eat more than you can lift.' – Miss Piggy

DREAMS, GOALS AND WANTS

This book gives you a lot of information and strategies to encourage your kids to eat more vegetables, but YOU have to use the knowledge and implement the techniques in order to make an actual change in your lives.

It is best to think about your aims in terms of basic day-to-day wants, longer-term goals and far-ranging dreams. It is easiest to start with wants (or perhaps just start with what you don't want).

WANTS

Each day, what do you want to see happen? If you have picked up this book, you may be in crisis mode, just trying to get through the day in one piece. Here are some examples of short-term wants. Feel free to grab from this list or adapt as suits:

- Get Junior to try one new vegetable this month.
- Aim to have recognizable (not hidden) vegetables on the dinner plate at least three nights per week.
- Make sure at least one snack per week contains vegetables.

GOALS

Looking to a longer period, say a month, a quarter or a year, what goals would you like to achieve when it comes to your family's healthy eating? Once you have stopped putting out fires, you may want to come up with a longer-term strategy to prevent them from occurring in the first place. For instance:

- Make a vegetable soup that everyone likes to eat.
- Buy some seeds and plant two or three types of vegetables in a small garden.
- Schedule a calm and happy family dinner that everyone attends at least once per week.

DREAMS

On a long-term basis, what sort of relationship with food would you dream up for your children? What is on your ultimate wish list? This may be too hard to contemplate right now, so I will tell you mine.

I aspire for my children to:

- say yes to food—to recognize foods and also try new foods if offered, eat a wide variety of foods and not be fussy;
- be able to (politely) say no to food—I do not want them to feel like they need to finish their plates or ask for seconds if they feel full;
- eat mindfully and with full presence most of the time;
- stop themselves from eating mindlessly—just because a desirable food is in front of them does not mean they need to eat it;
- understand their body signals and allow themselves to be comfortable with getting hungry;
- have the systems and techniques in place so they do not get too hungry and thus make poorer food choices (get hangry, take it out on others or eat everything in a five-mile radius);
- never eat emotionally (open up the fridge and pour all the contents down their throats), because they are bored or tired or for any other reason other than the fact that their bodies require some nutritious food;
- devour a treat gleefully on occasion with the utmost joy and no guilt;
- effortlessly select healthy, nutritious food from a wide variety of different sources because they inherently like to do so;
- know that I fed them vegetables consistently and persistently over the years because I LOVE them, and so I want them to treat themselves with as much love.

These may seem too momentous, but I have their entire lives (or the at least the first twenty years) to achieve these dreams. Bit by bit, with some focus, I know it is possible.

. . .

How to Implement Change

No matter how you look at it, you are trying to introduce changes to eating behavior, table manners and nutrition within your family. This could be a few small tweaks to improve things, a full overhaul of behaviors and mindset or something that falls in the spectrum between.

Regardless of how extensive the changes are, you need to work out the best route that comes with the least resistance. You want everyone to be on board so you sail smoothly through the rough seas, not start a mutiny against the captain of the ship.

So how do you get your resistant child to embrace the changes? Entire management textbooks have been devoted to this topic, and still many organizations get it wrong every day. The answer is that it depends. It depends on the extent of the changes, your child's personality and her ability to adapt to new situations. What is outlined below are the two alternative ways change can be handled.

Go Cold Turkey

State that from this date (say one week from now), this will be the new plan—three meals per day and two snacks, no eating between, vegetables first choice and freely available, etc. It will be like that from that date on. There is no going back. Perhaps this is good for certain behavior such as not being a short order cook anymore. You can declare that from this date forward there will be no alternative dinners.

Gradual Substitution

Alternatively, you can bring in the change more slowly. For instance, say that you are going to start with one family dinner all together per week. For this dinner, you are starting with a vegetable appetizer and then there will also be vegetables on your plate. Possibly one that you have not tried before. You do not have to eat it all, but it would be lovely if you would taste it.

Gradual substitution works especially well when you want your kids to try something new. Introduce a new vegetable in tiny amounts, find a vegetable similar to the one you are introducing (in taste, color or texture) and serve them together. Try for, say, one new vegetable per week. Taste buds change over time, so this method works well with our biology.

As noted earlier, health guru Dr. Libby Weaver states that you should aim to **double** the amount of plant food you currently eat, but she also advises to do this gradually. We eat 35 meals a week, so aim to add one more 'real food' meal each week for the next two months. If we only have, say, seven healthy meals at the start, then in two months this can double to 15. In a couple of months, DOUBLE the amount of nutrients are being introduced.

LOVE AND HEALTH

Imagine a world where people love their bodies and treat them with kindness and respect. Imagine if everyone knew when they were full and could say no to more food. Imagine if everyone had a natural curiosity toward new foods and were excited about giving them a try. We are born with all these innate abilities and they slowly erode away. Let's instead enhance them in our children and give them the lives they deserve.

Of course one little book like this is not going fix up every nuance to attain all these lofty aspirations. But maybe, just maybe, it could help with getting us a few steps along the path toward these wants, goals and dreams.

You may not be successful in getting broccoli past their lips every day, but you do have control over the overall attitude, behavior and culture in your family toward healthy eating. You are the leader and the gatekeeper for health and vitality. Use your knowledge and power for good.

It takes habits and schedules, commitment and energy, plus a little bit of fairy dust every single day. This is about LOVE and it is about HEALTH, and what else is more important? You have about 20 years to master this.

Start today.

8

THE 'HEALTHY' RECIPE

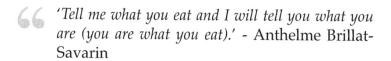 *'Tell me what you eat and I will tell you what you are (you are what you eat).'* - Anthelme Brillat-Savarin

RECIPE FOR SUCCESS

How can we implement our wants, goals and dreams around healthy eating? The seven 'ingredients' in the 'H-E-A-L-T-H-Y' acronym below help busy parents encourage their kids to eat and love vegetables. Each 'ingredient' has three or more strategies that have been proven to help coach even the fussiest eater out of unhealthy behaviors.

Some strategies are direct, and some are not. Some take a short time, and some involve a bit more effort. But together they provide a successful recipe for healthy eating. The best part is you don't even have to use all the ingredients and strategies to make vast strides toward vitality in your family. Choose a couple of techniques that you can implement easily and quickly with your little ones, and once you are happy with those, pick more.

Each of the ingredients are explained in detail in the next few chapters, but here is the basic outline:

H-E-A-L-T-H-Y Ingredients

Habit – create habits around eating vegetables

Encourage Variety – get a wide variety of vegetables into your kids

Accept and Allow – allow your children to understand their own bodies

Lay Down the Law – add some structure and routine around mealtimes

Talk – communicate with your kids

Hide 'Em– hide vegetables in meals and snacks

Yummy Fun – inject some FUN back into the kitchen

Start Cooking!

What are you waiting for? Dive in. It's best to follow the recipe in order, but please start somewhere. Don't delay in cooking up your own 'H-E-A-L-T-H-Y' recipe today.

9

HEALTHY INGREDIENT ONE (H) – HABIT

> 'Good habits formed at youth make all the difference.' - Aristotle

MAKE VEGETABLES AVAILABLE

The number one best thing you can possibly do to get your kids to eat more vegetables is to make them part of meals and have them available to eat every day in your home.

That is it.

I know it seems too easy or too boring or that it would never work.

It works.

Think of why your kids want to drink Coca-Cola or eat McDonald's or get the latest toy. Because they are constantly bombarded with visuals, media and advertising that encourages it. So do the same with vegetables in your household. Make vegetables a visible, accessible and natural part of the daily routine.

Do you find it stressful to brush your teeth? NO! You just do it. It's just something that gets done, that you do every day. As busy parents, we have to make dozens of food decisions each day. So creating habits and thus removing some of these is good for our mental health, as well as our family's physical health.

MAIN HABIT STRATEGIES

There are three main strategies that work for getting the kids to have an ingrained belief that vegetables are a normal part of daily life. These are:

- Always there
- Lead with vegetables
- Vegetables at every meal (even breakfast!)

ALWAYS THERE

Start with clearing out your kitchen cupboards, pantry and fridge of all the junk and packaged food (or put it on a high shelf). Only have healthy food in your family's line of sight. Children cannot drive to the store and buy chocolate, soda and cookies themselves, so while they are at home, they have to eat what is actually there.

Encourage your children to reach for vegetables (or fruit) as a first call if they are hungry. It is up to you whether they can go and grab a healthy option or ask you first. See the 'Lay Down the Law' chapter for more here. The point is to have vegetables and fruit readily available.

Chop up vegetables, wrap them in a damp paper towel and place in a plastic bag or humidity-controlled section of fridge. Having a fruit bowl sitting on the counter with some in-season, fresh fruit readily available is an enticing and healthy start.

If your child still says he is hungry and another carrot stick snack is not going to suffice, then encourage him to munch his way through an apple (cut it up and take off the skin for very young children). Just the act of eating it will take up some time before a proper meal is ready.

LEAD WITH VEGETABLES

Do you want the simplest, fastest and easiest technique to get your kids to eat more vegetables? Ta, da, da, da, da— here it is… are you ready?

Serve them some vegetables first.

Before 'the main course'. Yes, that is it. This is the number one best method to dramatically increase vegetable consumption.

Cut up one, two or three types of raw vegetables you already know they like, put them on a plate and say 'lunch (or dinner) is served'. It is part of the meal. There are so many benefits to this I am not sure where to begin. First, they are sitting at the table or at the kitchen counter and already eating, so you can keep an eye on them while you finish cooking. Second, eating vegetables is not overwhelming as there are only a few small selections on a plate. Third, the vegetables are not all put with the main course and therefore easily ignored for the more desirable parts.

Mama Tip - I often give them carrot sticks while I am making dinner, to tide them over and also ensure a vegetable has been eaten even before we sit down. – Marianne

And—huge bonus—if you do add vegetables with the main plate as well, there is not as much worry whether they are eaten or not. But if they are—double awesome!

One study showed that when a raw carrot appetizer was served first to kids, the total vegetable intake went up 50%. The children in the study ate not only the first course, but also other vegetables served later in the meal AND more of them.

The vegetables don't have to be raw. They can be lightly steamed, microwaved, stir-fried, baked, oven roasted or even remain frozen. To help get them down (at least at first) add a dollop of natural yogurt, hummus, some other dip or ketchup on the side. Scatter some herbs or a tiny amount of grated cheese on top. See more on these flourishes to add desirability in the variety and fun chapters.

Mama Story - Grated cheese on the top of pretty much anything will get my kids to eat it. – Annabelle

Do this at the start of every lunch and dinner for which you and your kids are at home. Make sure it is timed so that they will come to the kitchen or dining room and eat the small platter of vegetables just before the main course is ready to serve. This crudités dish is effectively the first course, and there is a natural progression to the next course.

*Mama Tip – **'The Sacrificial Vegetable'** – For the*

vegetable appetizer, put three vegetables on the plate, one of which is less favored. For example, cut up some capsicum, celery and radish. Place the plate out and wait for the 'Oh but I don't like radish'. All you say, is 'You don't have to eat it'. And then your darling munches on the other two vegetables. What just happened is your child happily ate two portions of vegetables. As Meatloaf says "two out of three ain't bad". And you never know, one day, the previously disliked vegetable may even be tried and eaten. – Julie

Vegetables at Every Meal

Incorporate vegetables into every meal. Every meal you say? Breakfast? Snacks? Dessert? Well maybe not every meal, every day (probably not ever in dessert) but yes, as much as you can when you are at home.

Between vacation time, Halloween, Christmas and a multitude of kids' birthday parties, I would say at least 10% of the year is taken up with the opportunity to eat junk or treat food. On top of that, you may not have much control over what your child eats when she is in childcare, school or when she visits friends and grandparents. So straight away you may only be able to influence 80% of her meals, and even the best parent skips some of those.

But don't despair, even a minuscule improvement in what your child is eating in terms of vegetables is fantastic. Start somewhere. One snack. Some vegetables on the plate at a couple of dinners per week. Any effort is better than nothing. You wouldn't be reading this book if you didn't want to try.

It may seem like a lot of hard work adding vegetables into lunch, dinner and snacks. I am not denying that it is a bit more effort, but it will significantly reduce your stress levels.

A common scenario in many households with children is absolutely no vegetables in any meals throughout the day and then they show up on the plate with the rest of the meal at dinner. The child is likely to bypass the vegetables and go directly for the good stuff—the meat or other type of protein and the potatoes, rice or other carbohydrate. Those few stems of broccoli are looking even more wilted and unappetizing by the time most of the meal is eaten and are easily ignored.

Then you, the awesome parent you are, think, wow, my little one hasn't had any vegetables at all today. Your requests turn into a spiral of doom of pleading or bribing or even threatening. Sound familiar? Sound stress inducing? Why do we put ourselves through this?

The alternative is a much more proactive, relaxed and happy approach. Throw some vegetables down before the main course at lunch and dinner, and then add a few more vegetables on the plate with the main course. Any snack should include a couple of bites of a favorite vegetable. Then by the time you all get to the main dinner meal, so what if the broccoli is forgotten? Your tiny human has already had her vegetable quota scattered throughout the day.

The key to this is to only put a **very small** amount in front of your child. I am talking two or three tiny stalks of broccoli, half a carrot chopped up, a few slices of cucumber, one small celery stick—and that is at each sitting, not all at once.

And it is fine if he doesn't eat it all, or that he eats only a few bites—**it's the habit of eating it every single day that counts**.

Mama Story - We serve at least two types of vegetables on Henry's dinner plate each night. This way he usually decides to eat at least one out of the two. There is less fighting. Plus, as a bonus, it is normal for him to see two vegetables on his plate. – Kay

The other main thing to remember is to be consistent. No backsies. You start this thing and continue. Make sure you are stocked with at least one or two vegetables you know he will eat and then you can add something he hasn't tried, or has and rejected before as well. More on this in the next chapter.

Just keep serving up vegetables—as an appetizer, as part of the main meal, or mixed in (much more about this in the 'Hide 'Em' chapter). Don't get discouraged. Be a parent. Be persistent. You can think of this new habit as a fantastic, healthy change or a way of wearing your child down, whatever helps.

Not sure where to start? The next few pages offer some scrummy ideas, and then check out the recipes section for some delicious favorites.

VEGETABLES AT BREAKFAST

Although you really do not have to offer vegetables at breakfast, why not? Is there something in your belief system that is holding you back from serving up vegetables at breakfast?

To add a little bit of green into a traditional breakfast, it is easiest to start with eggs. Add a bed of wilted spinach to a poached egg or throw some mushrooms, tomato and spinach into an omelet or breakfast frittata. With bagels or English breakfast muffins, spread some cream cheese and offer slices of avocado and tomato on top. Or simply have avocado on toast—great with a tiny smattering of salt and pepper. Get into the smoothie or juicing trend and throw some spinach into your next banana-berry concoction. Or go all out and follow other cultures that have vegetable soups, rice and vegetables or a selection of salad vegetables with cheese and bread at breakfast time (also see 'Backwards Day' in the 'Yummy Fun' chapter). At the very least, offer a bit of fruit on top of your child's cereal in the morning—chopped banana, peaches from a can or a handful of frozen berries warmed up make a delicious addition.

Vegetables at Lunch and Dinner

You have already presented a vegetable appetizer, so how to introduce them into the main event? You do not have to be fancy—you can put the very same vegetables that you had in the first course as part of the main course, maybe the cooked instead of raw version. Many children love and thrive on repetition and familiarity, and if it works and they still want to eat the same vegetables, then why not?

If a change is needed, then some new ways of presenting vegetables could be as a soup, wrapped in a rice paper or a tortilla, baked in the oven with a little bit of grated cheese melted on top, or finely sliced into a coleslaw. Or you can have some fun and make faces or scenes on the plate. See the 'Yummy Fun' and 'Recipes' chapters for more ideas.

Daddy Story – We often ask the kids what vegetables they want with dinner but only give them a choice of two or three. This gets their buy in to eating vegetables as they have had some control over the decision-making. So we say – do you want steamed broccoli or coleslaw with the chicken tonight? Just be prepared that each kid will give you a different answer – so maybe take turns with these 'choices'. – Mick

VEGETABLES AS SNACKS

Remember packaged snack foods marketed to kids are brightly cultured and cute, so you need to counter this with your own 'marketing' when designing snacks that involve vegetables.

Luckily, as you can eat them raw, they transport well and there is such a variety that vegetables, by their very nature, make ideal snack foods. Make sure there is a bit of carbohydrate, protein, fat or some of at least one of these three elements included with the vegetables in the snack. Think of snacks like mini-meals. They need to sustain your little ones until the next time they eat.

Here are some my guaranteed favorites:

- Carrot sticks with hummus or another type of dip
- Celery with some cut up cheese or peanut or almond butter
- Corn chips with fresh made avocado dip or guacamole

- A cup of vegetable soup (warmed up from the freezer)
- Warmed up edamame (takes two minutes from the frozen package)

As Easy as Brushing Your Teeth

The whole point of the 'Habit' approach is to make eating vegetables normal, expected and as effortless as brushing your teeth. Familiarity and frequency is the antidote to fighting, tears and rejection. Forming habits is a long-term strategy that is not flashy, but it gets results, and isn't that what being a parent is all about?

This strategy makes it easy to get the familiar vegetables eaten, but what if you want Junior to try something new? Find out the best ways in the next chapter.

ACTION ITEM

Present a small platter of vegetables as an appetizer before the main course at dinner tonight.

10

HEALTHY INGREDIENT TWO (E) – ENCOURAGE VARIETY

66 *'Maybe broccoli doesn't like you either.'* – Unknown

VARIETY IS THE SPICE OF LIFE

Having vegetables freely available and as the first choice for meals and snacks is the single best method to getting the whole family to consume more vegetables overall. But what if you want your kids to try something new? How do you get your little one (or indeed anybody) to try a new food?

MAIN 'ENCOURAGE VARIETY' STRATEGIES

There are three main strategies that help children to become more adventurous eaters. These are:

- Exposure
- Embrace the inherent variety in vegetables

- Present vegetables in different ways or in different settings

EXPOSURE

'Exposure' sounds complicated and scientific, but it is actually very easy. Put a tiny amount of the food you want your child to try on a plate and encourage her to taste it. Then over time, do it again and again and again.

That is it.

I know it seems too easy or too boring or that it would never work.

It works.

IT NOT ONLY WORKS, BUT IT HAS THE BACKING OF SCIENTIFIC studies that show it is the **single most effective method of adding variety into a person's diet**. Forget fun plates and hiding vegetables (although they will be discussed later), this is it.

The first step is to put a vegetable on your child's plate that he has either not eaten before or has refused to eat in the past. Put a tiny amount—a few peas, a couple of stalks of broccoli, a few pieces of carrot.

Then talk to your child and tell him that there are a couple of pieces of broccoli on his plate. You can explain that it is green like the peas he likes or tastes a bit like the cauliflower he tried last week. It helps to associate the new vegetable with something your child already finds familiar. Do not tell him it is healthy or good for him.

Remain neutral. The new vegetable is there and can be eaten.

> *Daddy Tip - You may want to temporarily invent a new name for the vegetable, if there's a stigma attached to the old name in the kid's mind. A colleague of mine had a story about referring to peas as 'green corn' for years with their children. – James*

Also tell him your expectations. This depends on how often your child has experienced the vegetable, how old he is and a number of other factors like how he copes with change. You can tell him that he does not have to eat it, or swallow it, but you would like him to taste it or take a bite. He can even pick it up with his hands, lick it or simply sniff it. Decide on what is acceptable and what is likely to bring out the best outcome for you and your child. Let him proceed at a pace that is comfortable for him, even if it seems glacial to you.

> *Mama Story - Alicia....she isn't as adventurous. She is reluctant to try new things but we still put them on her plate and ask her to try. If she doesn't we don't force it. – Zoe*

Children experience food differently from adults in that there is more of an experimental approach. It is not just the taste that is important, but also the shape, color, texture, look, smell and feel of the vegetable. The result of his exploration will help him to decide if tasting is an option. Utilize his natural curiosity, but don't ruin it. At the first outing, your child is likely not to try it. Remember that it does not matter if he screws up his face in disgust or even tries it and says 'I don't like it'.

The key to the exposure technique is to **repeat** your efforts. Every couple of days, or once a week, the particular vegetable is on your child's plate. How many times? Try **10 to 20** times before giving up. If there has been no progress after numerous attempts, try a different vegetable under the exposure strategy and then come back to the previous one at a later date. It is likely, after dozen times, or over the course of a month or two that your child will just start to eat the vegetable. It has become a normal fixture on his plate and the familiarity of seeing it all the time will lead to the action of trying it out and then eating it.

> *Mama Tip – All I would say is keep presenting. I was determined for Toby to eat broccoli due to its high nutritional content and because I like it so much so we always have it in the house. I put it on his plate every day for three months and he didn't touch it, or he might have tried a bit of it but didn't eat it. Then one day he picked it up and ate it. Toby has been eating it regularly ever since without complaint. I haven't had to do that with any other vegetable as he will eat pretty much anything now. – Zara*

Yes I know, it's a boring way to get new vegetables into your child. It is a lengthy process and there is no guarantee it will work. But sometimes parenting is a long-term game. You have nothing to lose and so much to gain, so try it.

> *Mama Story – If there is something new in season, we invite the twins to the kitchen and put a couple of bites on a plate and ask them to taste it. This is separate from meals and snacks. It makes it seem like a bit of an occasion. We get them to tell us what it reminds them of,*

what it smells like to them and to describe the texture or taste (crunchy, sweet). We tried it with artichokes the other day. Izzy said they were tasty, Caleb said they were horrible. They love giving their input. – Raquel

Why or how does it work? Scientifically it has been proven in various studies that small amounts of repeated tasting does change dislike to like as our tastes change and adapt over time. This is reinforced by our biology—did you know that each of our taste buds is replaced every two weeks?

From a parent standpoint, a child's willingness to eat anything is not just directly related to whether she likes the taste. It can depend on anything from the sight, smell and texture of the food to what she has already eaten that day, how tired she is and what kind of mood she is in.

Daddy Tip - If they are refusing a lot of foods, consider textures, particularly for kids who have sensory issues (e.g. don't like scratchy clothes / loud noise / bright lights). It may be that they dislike squishy foods, or some other particular texture. Try serving the same vegetable in a different way. – James

The other reason it works from a parental point of view is that you are embracing your child's inherent need to learn from repetition. Repetition can be the bane of our existence when we have to read the same bedtime story over and over, but it can be used to your advantage here. Repetition is the main way to reduce resistance. Yes, we heard it already in the Habits chapter: persistence really is the key to getting more vegetables—and a wider variety of them—into our children.

• • •

EMBRACE THE INHERENT VARIETY IN VEGETABLES (...OR Don't)

After reading the 'Exposure' strategy, you may be thinking that you would rather cut your losses—your kid likes peas and carrots and sometimes will even deem it worthwhile to eat some broccoli. You have three vegetables under your belt, why rock the boat?

Many books and articles state that you MUST get your child to eat a wide variety of food, but for busy fatigued parents, all we want to know is if there are a handful of vegetables that I know that my child will eat, is it okay to present them to him again and again?

The answer is of course it is! Your child should eat a wide of variety of foods, from the major food groups—some carbohydrate, protein and fat as well as fruit and vegetables. That way she is likely to gain the key nutrients she needs. However, within the category of vegetables, you don't have to get her to try and like everything. It is almost impossible to do so. Did you know that you could get your daily requirement of vitamin C just from eating a carrot and a handful of strawberries?

The most important thing is to get her to see eating vegetables—any vegetables—as a normal thing, part of the daily routine. Hence why establishing vegetables as a habit comes first. A secondary goal is to get her to love a bit of variety in her meals and become a more adventurous eater.

A repetitive but nutritious diet is perfectly acceptable. Children like predictability and routine so use that to your advantage. Stay on the tried and true and be happy with your decision.

Mama Story - I found that the kids would often want one thing for a week or two. So carrots, for instance, every day for a week. Or peas. Or corn. But all day, every day, day after day. You'd think they'd tire of it, but my kids liked a consistent run of something until they decided to try something else. – Annabelle

However...

Now let's try on the other hat. It is also a great idea to try to get your child to embrace the interesting, new and different. This may seem like I am negating everything that was just written, but in fact, the two ways of approaching vegetable intake can be complementary.

Perhaps your child is a bit sick, had a busy week or has some other changes in his life. Then do not add a new vegetable to the mix. But if your child is healthy, well rested and feels in a secure place, then what have you got to lose?

The great thing with vegetables is their inherent nature lends itself to variety. There is a huge assortment of different types of vegetables. Peas, corn, carrots and eggplant could not be more different from each other in taste, color, smell and texture. Next, different vegetables are best eaten seasonally – think of pumpkin in the fall and avocado in the summertime.

There is a large variety of color in vegetables, and this can be an advantage. So what if your little one turns her nose up at anything green? For now, invite him to eat yellow, orange and red instead. To be honest, the advice to 'eat the rainbow'—five different colors of fruit and vegetable —every day (or even every week) sounds exhausting to me, but some families and children love it. A spectrum of colorful vegetables gives you more chance to attain every single one of the nutrients that keep your body at its optimum level of health.

And there is always some type of vegetable that seems new or different, even to us grownups. Why not try purple cauliflower as a whole family, or incorporate the leaves from celery in a soup? Young children will sometimes try new things because they have not yet learned that they 'shouldn't' eat it. This is discussed more in the gardening section, but here are two words that can really up the ante in the interesting stakes—'edible flowers'.

PRESENT THE VEGETABLES IN DIFFERENT WAYS

If having a huge variety of vegetables—from freshly podded peas, to crunchy carrots, juicy sweet corn or smooth avocado—still does not create enough excitement, then how you cook, prepare and present the vegetables may well do the trick.

You do not have to do anything extra complicated. In fact you do not even have to cook vegetables. Little kids absolutely love eating frozen peas. Throw a few in a bowl and watch their pincer grip improve in the process. As an added bonus, frozen vegetables are proven to be as nutritious as fresh, as most are flash frozen at the time of picking.

Mama Story - Adam will eat cucumber and frozen peas (still frozen, no good if thawed). – Terri

There are so many different ways of cooking and preparing vegetables, so what is guaranteed to work? It can be a bit trial and error here, but look at it as a fun experiment. Try combining vegetables together. Some kids will dig into coleslaw and others will not touch it. Or cook them in an unusual way. If you usually present broccoli raw or steamed, why not try stir-frying it, or even baking it?

Mama Story - I made a raw vegetable salad with carrots and beetroot, and added cacao nibs. Told them it was a pink salad with chocolate chips. They both ate it, but picked stuff out. I'm pretty sure it was the lemon in the dressing that they weren't keen on. – Marianne

Maybe your child tells you he doesn't like spinach. Why not present it three different ways and then ask him if he really does not like it. Give it to him beneath a poached egg in the morning, blended into a smoothie at lunch and stuffed into cannelloni at dinner.

Or add some other flavors to the vegetable dish. You want your little one to recognize and like vegetables in their purest form, but additional flavor can enhance a dish and make it seem more desirable.

Mama Tip - Instead of serving meat and potatoes/pasta in a sauce with boring vegetables on the side, add a bit of sauce or flavor to the vegetables and serve the meat and carbohydrates in a more 'boring' style. That way the vegetables are yummy / interesting by comparison. – Emma

Use any of the following techniques:

- flavor on the side—ketchup, BBQ sauce, sweet chili, hummus, dips

- flavor as a covering—white sauce, cheese sauce, gravy
- flavor on the side or covering—salad dressing, mayonnaise, yogurt, sour cream
- jazzed up—use a squeeze of lemon, salt and pepper, fresh or dried herbs or a little grated cheese
- covered—battered, floured (with herbs), egg and bread crumbed

Mama Tip - Occasionally I let them have BBQ or tomato sauce (ketchup) on their vegetables. I make the sauce but keep it in the store bought bottle so they don't know the difference. – Sally

Daddy Story – I don't cook that often but when I do, I sometimes make 'gourmet broccoli' – steamed broccoli with a sprinkling of herbs, a drop of red wine and grated cheese on top. The whole family loves it. – Rob

You may have noticed that your child may want the same vegetable for dinner when you are at home, but if you are out at a big family picnic at the park she will happily try something that is a bit different. What is that all about? What has happened is that she is already out of her comfort zone, so she may continue with eating outside of her comfort zone.

A particularly cool way to continue with this line of thought is to change other things in your child's life. If you want him to try new foods, then get him to try and do other things that are different. For example, listen to different music, take him to a different playground or wear some new clothes.

Have enough structure in her life that she still feels secure, but change something else up—new karate class anyone? —and she may just eat that cauliflower you have been placing on her dinner plate.

There is an absolute ton of ideas around this concept, and this section is meant to pique your interest, to start you thinking of the possibilities in your household.

We have spent the last two chapters discussing parent-led approaches to introducing vegetables. Now let's take a step back and get our children more involved in the decision-making.

ACTION ITEM

Buy a new vegetable that you have not eaten before (or at least not for a long time), and get the whole family involved in trying it. You never know, it could become a family favorite.

11

HEALTHY INGREDIENT THREE (A) – ACCEPT AND ALLOW

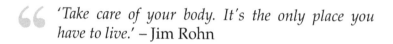

> *'Take care of your body. It's the only place you have to live.'* – Jim Rohn

RESPECT THEIR BODIES

You can lead a horse to water... so the saying goes. And you can provide your child with lovingly prepared and nutritious food, but you cannot make her eat it. There are very few things babies and very young children have complete control over, and what they put in their mouths and ultimately consume is one of them.

We know we cannot force feed, so we read books like this one. And there are tons of strategies in here that busy parents can employ that will make eating vegetables seem more desirable and easier to our children. But this chapter is more about getting out of our own way.

It is very important to:

- **Accept** that our little ones have control over eating decisions, and
- **Allow** our children to listen to their bodies.

This is a relatively short chapter, but it could prove to be the hardest one to understand and implement, because for many of us, listening to our bodies and mindful eating are abilities that we may have lost.

Main 'Accept and Allow' Strategies

There are three main strategies that allow our tiny humans control over their own bodies. These are:

- Follow Satter's 'Division of Responsibility'
- Reframe hunger
- Six magical little words—'You don't have to eat it.'

Satter's 'Division of Responsibility'

Lunch is ready. Your busy child runs to the table, gobbles down a few bites and then wants to leave again. You know he hasn't eaten enough. Then comes the begging, bribing and barking.

But look back at that decision—*you* decided that he had not had enough to eat, and then *you* decided to try and get a few more mouthfuls down his throat, ultimately ending in frustration and failure.

However, it is not up to you to decide whether he has had enough to eat.

Period.

But, you say, 'a hangry temper tantrum will occur in an hour's time' or 'he won't go for his midday nap if he is hungry' or 'it's just plain rude to leave the table'. For now, this does not matter. You will have in place some rules and structure around table manners and providing food after a meal is not eaten fully. The next chapter delves into all of that. But for now, it is his decision to eat or not to eat.

Ellyn Satter describes this in such an eloquent way that at first glance, it doesn't seem like feeding your children could be reduced to something so beautifully simple. However, when it comes to decisions around eating, we need to go back to basics. She recommends:

- The parent is responsible for what, when, where (of feeding).
- The child is responsible for how much and whether (of eating).

Refer to www.ellynsatterinstitute.org or her books for more detail.

If you follow this recommendation, then you, as the parent, provide the nutritious food at the time when the child is expected to eat and at the location (e.g.: the kitchen table) where she is expected to eat it. Your little one will decide whether she will eat at all, and if so how much.

How this works in practice is to have relatively stable meal times, a known location to eat food and a way for your child to decide the 'how much' part. Whether you put food directly on her plate or let her serve herself, she decides how much to eat of the food that is provided.

There are always at least a couple of things you know she has liked and eaten previously.

Of course, there can be rules around this, like she must take at least a small amount of all the main types of food on offer. She can ask for seconds if there is some available. It is perfectly okay within the realm of giving them so much control to say things like, 'I will get you more pasta in a moment, but why don't you eat a couple of carrots'.

Mama Story – It's a bit of tough love in my house! I only cook one meal so if they decide they don't want to eat it that is fine, but they still must sit with us during dinner. They tend to end up eating at least a little of it. – Mandy

Your little ones will still need some help when it comes to sweets and desserts—it is not a free for all. For example, there is no seconds when it comes to servings of dessert. More on these suggested rules in the next chapter. With these rules in place, it is unlikely that your child will eat too much, but you may still be worried that she will not eat enough. Let's now take a look at this more closely.

REFRAME HUNGER

I can hear you howling from here. That is waaaaaaay too much control to give to my four-year-old! Given the choice, he will not eat anything and then be hungry. If he is hungry he will get angry (hungry-angry or 'hangry'). If he is hungry he will not sleep well. Hungry is bad. I am a bad parent.

It is time to reframe hunger and what it actually means. Making HUNGER = BAD is not helpful to any of us.

The first thing to note is that your child will not starve himself. Did you know an appropriate amount of food for one meal for a toddler is about a fistful? That is all. He may look like he is eating like a bird, but his intake is reasonable for his age. If he is sleeping well at night, has energy during the day, his skin and teeth look fine and he eats something from most food groups over the course of a week, then there is no indication that he is suffering from any ill effects of malnutrition or starvation. Take those negative thoughts out of your mind.

> *Mama Tip – I firmly believe that they will eat as much as they need. Some days they eat hardly a thing, and some days they eat heaps… it evens out in the end. – Terri*

Remember what this chapter is about—**allowing** our children to listen to their own bodies. Think how miraculous our human bodies are—we are born with the innate sense of deciding when we are full and also have an innate want for a healthy balanced diet that provides us with nutrition and energy.

And then we slowly learn to ignore our body signals. We get bombarded with fast food advertising. The average preschooler sees **three ads per day for fast food**. We are taught to finish whatever is on our plates or otherwise it is 'wasteful' or 'we won't get dessert'. This madness has to stop.

Talk to your children about the feelings of hunger and fullness and how they can be on a scale from very hungry to very full. At various times, before and after meals, get them to tell you if they are so hungry they feel sick or faint, very ready to eat, kind of ready to eat, not hungry, slightly satisfied, very satisfied or stuffed/very full. If they are younger, this can be shown in a visual form or explained with dolls. Get her to describe how her body feels, especially her stomach (tummy). When she says she is finished with a meal, ask her 'Are you still hungry or are you feeling full?' which is a much more neutral question than 'Are you full?'

Plus talk to your (older) children about things other than physical ('tummy') hunger such as taste or smell hunger (wanting to eat because you know you will love it) or emotional hunger (wanting to eat because you are bored or sad). Ask them what they could do instead of eating if they are not really hungry.

Mama Tip - Did you know a lot of people confuse hunger with thirst? Sometimes if your child says they are hungry they may instead need a big glass of water. If in doubt offer them one anyway. – Julie.

Overall, it is important to shift from a state of fear about hunger itself. If your child is hungry, that does not make you a bad parent. It is a normal and healthy state for a child (and adults as well).

Filling up your children on less than nutritious food because you are wary of them being hungry can do them more harm than letting them wait a bit for their next meal.

There are many upsides to hunger. You start to feel connections in your body, realize how your body can change its state, know what physical hunger feels like and learn to survive (wait out) short-term hunger. Feeling a bit hungry and waiting for a meal teaches patience, self-control and how to cope with frustration, all-important facets of an independent adult. Like fullness, hunger is not bad or good, it is just a different state that the body may be in.

Daddy Tip - In fact they 'should' be hungry when mealtime rolls around. That way they are more likely to eat the meal and enjoy it. I would recommend no snacks for an hour or so before a meal, at least. Like our grandmothers all used to say "you'll spoil your dinner". – James

SIX MAGICAL LITTLE WORDS - 'YOU DON'T HAVE TO Eat It'

So how does Satter's advice translate into real world parenting? Your six-year-old sits at the table, looks at the plate in front of him and says, 'Yuck'. Your toddler wants to scramble down from the table after two bites of food. Your pre-teen grumbles about having pasta again. What is your response? Your response is this. It is always this:

'You don't have to eat it.'

I wish I had known about this earlier and saved myself a few years of tears and stress. This strategy came from a great blog post from Leigh Anderson on scarymommy.com called 'Six Words That Are Guaranteed to End Picky Eating'. This was her suggestion after she read Satter's book:

'You don't have to eat it.'

Try it at the next mealtime and instantly recognize how great it feels to say those six magic words. Shoulders are lowered. Stress levels have plummeted. Remember, the next chapter deals with mealtime structures and table manners so that your child will eat something eventually and never get ridiculously hungry. So do not worry that your kid will never eat again. For this meal, right now, with your little boy who does not want the tomatoes in the salad on his plate, all you have to say is:

'You don't have to eat it.'

Mama Story - They just have to try it. I try not to make a big deal out if it - in my attitude and in my voice. "That's OK, you don't have to eat it if you don't like it. I just want you to try it." – Marianne

These six words will transform your dinner table, your stress levels and your life. Say it calmly, say it with a smile, and continue on with eating your own plate of delicious dinner.

'You don't have to eat it.'

FINAL WORDS ON ACCEPT AND ALLOW

Of course, you can lightly ask 'Are you sure you don't want a few more bites?', or 'Are you sure you are full?' or gently remind your kids that there will not be another meal for X amount of hours. But ultimately you have to accept their decisions about their own wee bodies.

Mama Story - We often make a game of it and use their age to encourage them to "eat two bites of broccoli because you're two!" or "eat five more peas because you're five!". When you think about the size of their tummy is the size of their closed fist, it's not that big, so we encourage it, but only lightly. – Annabelle

Self-regulation is a vital lifelong habit. Give yourself a break on this one—do not think you need to teach it. Get out of the way and let it develop in your children naturally.

ACTION ITEM

Practice saying in a calm manner with a smile on your face: "You don't have to eat it".

12

HEALTHY INGREDIENT FOUR (L) – LAY DOWN THE LAW

'*After a good dinner one can forgive anybody, even one's own relatives.*' – Oscar Wilde

GUIDELINES AROUND MEALTIMES AND EATING BEHAVIOR

Do you want the best chance of eating healthier as a family? Then one of the most important things to address has nothing whatsoever to do with actually consuming more vegetables. Instead focus on structure and routine, rules and guidelines, and valuing family meals together.

Deciding on and then emphasizing certain expectations around mealtime behavior has a lot of benefits. It makes everyone in the household feel secure to know that there is a set and predictable number of meal and snack times per day, and if they miss one, another meal or snack will be available later.

When everybody knows and agrees on the set guidelines it can reduce stress and arguments as it takes the emotion part away. And it brings the family together.

Regular family meals can actually be an enjoyable experience, but at the very least you can monitor intake of food, your child starts to learn some table manners and she will sit upright at the dining table, which aids good digestion. Overall, structure around meals, eating behavior and family meal times encourages more mindful eating, and that is one of our main long-term goals for our tiny humans.

Main 'Lay Down the Law' Strategies

There are three main strategies that create a structured and secure eating environment in the home. These are:

- A regular mealtime routine
- Behavior expectations and rules
- Family mealtimes together

A Regular Mealtime Routine

Children thrive in a predictable environment, so use that to your advantage and create a simple mealtime structure that can be adhered to. Of course this will not be possible every day, but having a basic routine is better than nothing at all.

So what is a good guideline for meal and snack times? Keep it as simple as you can so everyone in the family understands it easily. Three main meals per day, breakfast, lunch and dinner, placed around the same time each day (weekends may differ from weekdays). Two snacks are offered between these times. Remember snacks are like mini-meals and contain some vegetables (or fruit) plus a small portion of other food groups—carbohydrate, protein and fat (if possible). Some days you may not need one of these snacks. Sometimes you may also want to add a dessert, fruit or snack before bedtime. The time periods for each meal and snack are up to you and may change as your family grows, but a total of FIVE meals and snacks per day is a good place to start.

Mama Story – They have the standard five meals per day. If they don't eat much they get warned that lunch is not for a long time. I may still leave it on the table for them to come back to within ten minutes. Sometimes they just need to visit the smallest room in the house! - Sally

This type of structure ensures a child can listen to her own body and make decisions on whether and how much to eat based on her body signals of fullness and hunger as discussed earlier. Using this simple mealtime structure, there is no more than a three-hour gap during the day between meals, so there is no time to get overly hungry. It is a reasonable yet flexible schedule that is easy to learn and respect.

The point is to have some periods of the day when your family does not eat. As a parent you can decide on the appropriate response if your little one requests food at times other than those set. This depends on whether he seems particularly hungry, whether he missed eating at the prior allocated time (or didn't eat much of what was on offer) and how old he is. Some families implement a no snacking between times hard rule. After all, the next meal or snack may be as little as half an hour away. Other parents bring out the leftovers of what was not eaten at the prior meal and offer that. Still others offer something simple like an apple. Do what you think is best for you and your child while respecting the mealtime structure that is in place.

> *Mama Tip - Eating between meal and snack times can be a GREAT way to get vegetables into the kids. Have a container of raw carrot and celery sticks cut up in the fridge and they can be the 'between meals hungry time snacks'. A bowl of cherry tomatoes on the table, or raw things to dip in hummus. All good. – Annabelle*

After dinner, especially if not a lot of dinner is eaten, this can become a big issue. Ultimately, you want your child to eat a good portion of her dinner, but if that has not happened, there needs to be a plan in place for how you want to deal with that. Do you have a rule that there is no extra food if dinner is not eaten or offer something plain like a banana, fruit in natural yogurt or a cheese sandwich? It is not nice to go to bed hungry, but your child also needs to learn the new rules of your household. How you approach snacks and after dinner meals may change as your child grows.

> *Mama Story – I do leave their dinner that is not eaten till bedtime just in case they get hungry again so they can finish their dinner then. – Nora*

BEHAVIOR EXPECTATIONS AND RULES

Teaching and valuing good behavior around mealtimes indirectly creates an environment where more vegetable consumption is likely. Following rules in one area (mealtime behavior) leads to following instructions in another area (eating behavior). The two complement and reinforce each other. Plus, having table manners sets your child up to be an adult who gets invited back to places.

Select a handful of rules that are the most important to you and promote those. Choose ones that a small child will understand. There are a lot to choose from, so pick your favorites. Not too many of you will go nuts trying to remember and stick to them all.

Some examples:

- wash hands before meals
- respect meal and snack times
- say please and thank you
- sit down to eat (at the table or elsewhere)
- do not to talk with mouth full
- no toys, phones or TV watching at the dinner table
- wait until everyone has finished before leaving the table
- (or) ask nicely to get down from the table

No discussion of rules around eating would be complete without talking about rewarding with food, mostly of the sweet variety. Yes, candy, lollies, sweets, chocolate, lollipops, marshmallows, dessert, pudding. Whatever you call it and whatever you choose, sweet food has been used as a treat or reward by many a guilty, frazzled parent when they are just trying to get a pea to pass their child's lips. Who hasn't heard, "if you don't eat your vegetables you won't get any ice cream?"

If we are talking potty training over a limited amount of time, this may be okay. However, this is the biggest NO-NO of all for getting your child to eat more vegetables and should NEVER be used. Just because it is common, that doesn't make it the right thing to do. Take it off the table (literally) as an option.

If used it teaches your child that the treat food is 'better' than the vegetable that he is eating. It also may aid him to ignore bodily signals and finish his plate just so he can get a treat or dessert (see 'The Clean Plate Club' earlier). A sweet bribe can end up being associated with a happy outcome and so be emotionally fulfilling, not a linkage that should be made to attain the goal of a lifelong healthy relationship with food.

By all means, have dessert, but do not link it to what is eaten or not eaten for dinner. Some families choose to have rules around dessert, like it happens twice per week on set days. This allows some excitement and anticipation around dessert and also follows the predictable routine promoted in the first strategy.

Mama Tip - The girls get to choose treat night twice a week. Their choice of day and treat. – Deanna

I know you are swearing at me. I know this is hard. I do not expect anyone to be perfect at this. By all means reward eating a few more vegetables with a promise of a half hour of TV after dinner or to play with a special toy (occasionally), but NOT with sweet food. Remember your goals and stop using ice cream as a threat or bribe. Instead look forward to it as a Sunday night treat for the whole family that is enjoyed after dinner regardless of whether any broccoli was eaten at all.

Mama Story - Most children in the world have never tasted ice cream and frankly I think it would be rude not to eat it. – Terri

FAMILY MEALTIMES TOGETHER

It is hard to scramble a meal together at the end of the day and all eat as a family, but the benefits of having family mealtimes, at least a few times per week, are huge. If weekdays are too hard, try for Sunday dinner or even a weekend lunch. The point is to schedule in one or two unmissable, everyone is there, family meals. No TV on, no mobile phones or toys at the table. Just the family.

Family meals together do not have to be lengthy occasions. As little as 10 to 15 minutes, especially for toddlers and very young children, is enough. Aim for no longer than half an hour for weeknights.

Then try to make it fun and relaxed. I know it seems impossible, but imagine if a family meal were the highlight of everyone's day instead a chaotic mess? Imagine if they encouraged family bonding instead of growling, yelling and complaining. It can happen if you focus on it and if it is important to you. It doesn't matter what you talk about—discuss the food, the weather or current events. The fact that you are all eating together with nothing else presently interrupting or distracting everyone is the main point.

If you are still not sure what the big deal is, then note these benefits. Studies have found that family dinners are directly connected to ALL of the following:

- lower obesity rates

- better connection between family members
- reduced stress levels
- feelings of stability and security
- increased self-esteem in kids
- improved grades
- reduced incidence of substance abuse in teenagers
- AND this is amazing—family dinners have been shown to be better than reading aloud for building literacy in young children! (Yes, really).

Mama Story – Growing up, we always sat together as a family. I think this is very important so you can supervise eating habits, instill good manners and develop your relationship with your child around mealtimes. – Zoe

Now you are halfway through the book, and you may be wondering where the quick fixes and five-minute shortcuts for busy parents are. Sorry about that. Instead, I want you to SLOOOOOOOW down. Spend an afternoon cooking and baking with your little one. Have a leisurely dinner with the whole family. Take a bite of your delicious frittata, put your fork down and chew it thoughtfully. Slowing down helps a busy family—it decreases stress levels, adds some calm into everyone's day and allows you all to come together for a quick check in before bustling onto the next thing.

BEING FLEXIBLE IS THE KEY TO GOOD STRUCTURE

Does this seem like too much structure? Does it feel restrictive and limiting? Most parents say that it actually provides MORE freedom and less stress as everyone knows the main rules, and then you can decide on the less important parts.

In the fabulous and highly recommended book *French Children Don't Throw Food*, Pamela Druckerman notes a favorite paradox that in order for (French) parents to have authority, they should be saying 'Yes' most of the time. For example, your child wants to eat a teaspoon of honey at breakfast time. Within the framework that you have created, it is still a mealtime and your child has asked, so you should say 'Yes'. Or your kids want to have an ice cream straight after school instead of after dinner on a 'dessert' day. Great—allow them some control. Say 'Yes'. Laying down the law is about setting limits but also about observing your child and adapting to situations within the structure upon which you all agreed.

After habits, variety, accepting our own bodies and setting up routines and limits, you may be thinking, what could be left? Next up is one of the most important, but overlooked, aspects of eating success—communication.

ACTION ITEM

Set a date for at least one family dinner this week.

13

HEALTHY INGREDIENT FIVE (T) - TALK

66 'Don't worry that children never listen to you; worry that they are always watching you.' - Robert Fulghum

COMMUNICATION 101

In the last ingredient, 'Law Down the Law' of our 'H-E-A-L-T-H-Y' recipe, there was not a single tip that involved helping children to actually eat their greens. And again with 'Talk', not a lot of actual ingestion and digestion is directly involved.

However, there is immense value in communicating with your children about healthy eating, good table manners and vegetables in general. Whether they are two or twelve, they will understand you if you make your talk interesting, explain yourself clearly and repeat yourself often enough.

Some days it may not seem like much is going in, but it is. And even if your words are not landing, your actions and behavior sure are. They are sponges. Use that to your advantage.

> *Mama Tip – Talk to them about it. "This is an eggplant... can you say eggplant? Does it look like an egg? Do you think a chicken laid it? No? Then what a wacky name?" etc. – Sally*

It is really important to talk with your kids about the changes that are going to happen in your household. Notice I said talk WITH, not TO. Get their buy in, get their help. For example, you can say that vegetables will be first choice for snacks, that there will be no eating between meals and that there will always be some vegetables on their plates at dinner time. Then for the 'buy in' part, ask your kids what their favorite vegetables are, and start with those ones in the first week. Communication is the key to accepting change.

Main 'Talk' Strategies

There are three main communication strategies that improve the chances of your kids embracing the whole eating vegetables paradigm shift. These are:

- Praise and encouragement
- Embrace the inherent greatness of vegetables
- Model the behavior that you want

Praise and Encouragement

Nothing beats good old-fashioned praise to encourage the behaviors you want to have in your home. It's free, easy and always available. It helps to make eating vegetables not just a normal but an enjoyable experience for your little one. It should always be used before any other external incentive or reward, the go-to option at any and every opportunity.

Praise for trying. Say "Well done for picking up and licking that piece of parsnip, I know it seems a bit strange, like a pale carrot". Praise for succeeding—"Wow you ate all five beans on your plate tonight, what a big boy you are". Try to be as specific as possible—"Good on you for trying the salad with the nuts in it that Daddy made". Find something encouraging to say each day, even if it is not directly related to eating vegetables—"You used your knife and fork really well tonight".

Being encouraging can take many forms beyond talking to your child. This can include smiles, hugs, high-fives, clapping your hands or even doing a happy dance.

Some of you may think this is taking things too far. Kids should eat their vegetables and be happy that there is food on the table! You may find it a bit silly, even outrageous to heap praise on your offspring just because she is munching on a lettuce leaf. Maybe you are worried about starting something that is required each time greens are served up.

The first thing to remind yourself is that giving your kids a bit of praise for engaging in behaviors you want is not spoiling them, but in fact, just great parenting. Remember, it is a low-key incentive. Just because you say thank you or give your child a high five when he eats all his spinach does not mean you will have to do it each time. Compare that to rewarding him with chocolate or a toy for each bite of greens—then you are getting yourself into murky territory. Also, you choose your level of praise. Maybe a simple 'thank you' will suffice. But if you up the encouragement levels, so what? It is a MEANS to an END. An end where your child eats healthy in an effortless manner. At the very least, it brings a sense of positivity to dinnertime.

EMBRACE THE INHERENT GREATNESS OF VEGETABLES

It is time to get excited about vegetables and convey that to your tiny human. By showing just how great vegetables are when your kids are young, it becomes part of the wallpaper, an assumed and normal fabric of family life as the kids grow.

> *Mama Tip - I try to explain the importance of vegetables and how they help our bodies to function better – but in a kid friendly way. – Deanna*

Talk vegetables up. There are many ways to approach this.

Already we have talked about using the 'What's In It For Me (WIIFM)' approach to touting the benefits of vegetables (see the Benefits chapter). Use some of those examples. Yes vegetables are good for you, but that is too boring and too general. Get interesting and get specific. Inject short conversations about why vegetables are not only important but really cool into daily life.

Did you know that *The Guinness Book of Records* lists avocado as the most nutritionally complete fruit in the world? How amazing is that?

Mama Tip - I tell my girls that their eyes sparkle when they eat green food. This includes lots of overacting, shielding my eyes from theirs and even putting sunglasses on etc. Works a treat. – Mandy

Use the five senses. For instance, show your kids just how many different colors of vegetables there are. Make it a game to tell you the color of the vegetables when you are at the store. Create a coleslaw, salad or vegetable platter with as many different colors of produce as you can get. Another time, discuss texture and feel—pop peas out of their pods, strip off corn from the cob, break a snap pea in half, squish a cherry tomato between your fingers. Or get them to notice the different smells—for instance compare raw to roasted pumpkin. Notice that I have not even discussed tasting the vegetables. For now, you are getting your kids excited about them in other contexts.

Mama Story - My kids love it when we do 'Color Dinner Week'. We had 'Monday Green Night' so everything on plate had to be green (meat was still normal color with green sauce and green vegetables with it). Next night was a different color. This is also a great way to get them to try new foods. – Nora

Is this forcing vegetables onto your kids or marketing them too hard? Are you being too 'tricky'? There are some answers to these objections. First, just do what appeals to you—you may love getting your kids to learn their colors better, or want to cook something in an unusual way. Or perhaps you haven't opened a pea pod since you were a child and want to try it again after so many years. Second, what is not to love about this? It is fun, easy, cheap and gets your kids interested in vegetables. And so what if there is a bit of marketing or trickery involved? Every day, your child gets bombarded with media messages that advertise junk food as a normal and great thing to eat. You are doing your part to somewhat offset these messages. You are not ever going to go too 'big', unless you commission a billboard flashing up salad ideas outside your house.

MODEL THE BEHAVIOR THAT YOU WANT

Perhaps you get the feeling your kids don't want to hear your latest fun fact about avocado. Fine. Don't talk. Communicate in other ways.

Being a good role model is part of being a good parent. So model the behaviors you want to see in your child. Always have a taste of something new and try to say something positive or at a least neutral about it. Please don't screw up your face and say 'Yuck'—you are a grown up, and you are better than that.

Have vegetables on your plate and eat them with your meal. Choose some carrot sticks with hummus as a snack, or cut up an apple to share. And for goodness sake, do not grumble or complain if someone else in the household has made a meal that you dislike. If you are not going to eat it, you can still at least pick at it while your child is in the room. There will usually be something on your plate you like, so eat that first.

Daddy Tip - Let the kids try a bite of a new vegetable from your plate, even if it's something you don't think they'll like. That way it is perceived as a treat or a privilege to eat it, and there's no pressure if they don't like it. – James

Try not to say 'I don't like pumpkin' or 'I have never liked Brussels sprouts'. This allows your children to identify with disliking a particular vegetable and makes it even harder to get them to actually try it themselves.

Overall, make sure your attitude conveys a love of healthy food, the ability to choose food wisely and pleasure in mealtime rituals.

RINSE AND REPEAT

The value of repetition has already been discussed, but, well, it is worth repeating. Repetition is how we learn. Repetition is how habits are formed. Communicating with your child with encouragement, describing how great vegetables are and modeling desired behaviors are all easily repeatable tasks that create positive results.

Now let's move back into actually cooking for our kids and consider the merits and warnings around hiding vegetables.

ACTION ITEM

Heap an extraordinary amount of praise onto your child for some desired behavior at dinner tonight (however small) and notice the response.

14

HEALTHY INGREDIENT SIX (H) – HIDE 'EM

'Vegetables are a must on a diet. I suggest carrot cake, zucchini bread, and pumpkin pie.' - Jim Davis

HERE IS YOUR PERMISSION SLIP TO HIDE VEGETABLES

You are **allowed** to hide vegetables in your kids' food. Of course, your little ones need to learn to see how vegetables look in nature and to like the taste of them as they are.

However, hiding them is a great alternative and complementary technique to get vegetables (and their vital nutrients) into your children without a fuss.

Understandably, you don't want to undo any good work already started in making eating vegetables a habit. You certainly don't want to have to rely on this (sometimes more labor intensive) method to get nutrients into your little ones. And you want your child to know what a carrot looks like. So why do it?

First, this method gets vegetables (and therefore all the goodness and nutrients that come with them) into our child. Second, it gets them without much conflict, fuss or even noticing, especially on days when you cannot face another dinnertime battle. Third, it is relatively easy to grate, puree or mash some vegetables into a favorite family dish after you have done it a few times. And it can actually be quite fun and a nice alternative to the other strategies in this book.

And remember, this is a complementary strategy—not something to be used every day. You can use it instead of OR as well as getting your child to eat fresh or cooked vegetables in the purest form. For example, you could have a pureed vegetable soup at lunch and then at dinner go for the 'courses' approach with a raw vegetable starter. Or at dinner you could produce spaghetti bolognaise with a ton of hidden vegetables in it with a small salad on the side.

Main 'Hide 'Em' Strategies

There are three main strategies for hiding vegetables. These are:

- Hide vegetables in 'normal' dishes
- Hide vegetables in plain sight
- Hide vegetables in cakes and treat foods (WARNING!)

HIDE VEGETABLES IN 'NORMAL' DISHES

There is a full spectrum of hiding methods, best vegetables to use (color and texture can play a big part) and types of recipes in which vegetables are most to least invisible.

Here are some ways to hide vegetables from most to least disguised:

- pureed/blended
- mashed
- grated
- chopped up small
- covered/ wrapped

The easiest way to cook vegetables so they are can be pureed or mashed is to boil, steam, roast or microwave them until soft. If your little one still won't touch anything green, then focus on vegetables that are not bright in color that can be concealed well such as cauliflower, parsnip, butternut, zucchini and squash.

The best place to start is in dishes that naturally lend themselves to having vegetables almost invisible in them. Here are some main food types that are easy vegetable concealers:

- pureed/blended—smoothie, soup, vegetable dip, mac 'n' cheese
- mashed—curry, pie, combined with mashed potato
- grated—pasta, scrambled eggs, omelet, fritters
- chopped up small—pasta, fried rice, frittata, soup, stew, casserole, or on pizza/in sushi (hidden in plain sight—see more on this below),

- covered/wrapped—Asian style rice wraps, Mexican style wraps, battered, bread crumbed (see hidden in plain sight below)

Some recipes can have more than one type of hidden vegetable. Our family's recipe for spaghetti bolognaise has a small amount of ground beef (mince) plus at least SIX types of vegetables in various forms. Usually it includes grated carrot, chopped onion, diced pepper and celery, shredded spinach, plus a can of pureed tomatoes. See the Recipes chapter for the full recipe.

Please note that by no means should this stop you from putting at least one visible vegetable on the table at lunch and dinner. Your little one needs to get used to seeing vegetables on the table.

Worth noting is that giving vegetables in a pureed, soup or smoothie form comes with its own set of negative implications. It is important for toddlers (and older children) to work out that food needs to be bitten and chewed on, that food can be different textures and some of those will be hard and crunchy. If foods are dished up mostly soft (or drinkable in the case of smoothies) then they won't learn about texture in the same way. Even more importantly, a continuous diet of soft foods means that their bodies may not learn to digest food properly. Chewing stimulates the digestive system and sets the body up to retain the best nutrients from the food eaten. Smoothies and soups can be a great part of your family's diet, but don't rely on them.

Making vegetables invisible involves an art of deception. This may not sit well with some of you, so after a while, it is within the rules of the game to tell your kids what hidden nutrition is in their meals. Be sneaky and then stop being sneaky. Or, as you will see in the next section, allow them to see, or even help you, with vegetable camouflage.

HIDE VEGETABLES IN PLAIN SIGHT

Disguising vegetables does not always have to involve blending them so they are completely invisible. Finely chopping, grating, coating or wrapping vegetables can effectively disguise vegetables in plain sight.

What is so great about this strategy is that you do not even have to be that tricky about it. Give a kid some pieces of pepper, tomato and mushroom on a plate and he could turn his nose up at it. Put the same thing on slice of pizza with some melted cheese on top and it will disappear before your eyes.

Even better—get them to help you. They can place the chopped up pieces on the pizza, or inside the sushi rolls. They can help you egg and breadcrumb the cauliflower or broccoli ready for roasting. And then they will eat it.

Mama Tip - I do have a delicious zucchini (courgette) cake recipe. It's not done for hiding though. The kids like to help make it. – Sally

Kids are funny beings—if you invite them to grate zucchini (watch carefully little fingers with the grater) and then toss it into the scrambled eggs they are even more likely to eat it than if you served it up the eggs with the hidden vegetables in it without their assistance.

Mama Story – A few years back, before my own baby was born, I looked after my niece and nephew one night.

Their parents told me that they were unlikely to eat any vegetables so just make something fun or get takeaways. I took this as a challenge. I had grown a lot of spinach in our back garden, so I lightly steamed it and then blended it into mashed potatoes, making the potatoes bright green. My niece and nephew saw every step I did, gobbled up this cool bright green mash, and asked for more. – Pearl

Sometimes, hiding chopped vegetables in say pasta or fried rice becomes a game. My son loves finding a piece of pepper in amongst the penne. He has been known to ask for more pasta just so he could 'find' the bits of vegetables and eat them.

HIDE VEGETABLES IN CAKES AND TREAT FOODS (WARNING!)

Vegetables can be hidden in cakes, muffins, loaves and other sweet treats, but please enter this territory carefully. As noted, hidden vegetables exist on a spectrum. A six vegetable spaghetti bolognaise is at one end, and a full chocolate cake with a single parsnip grated in falls at the other.

It is very important NOT to keep vegetables hidden solely in sweet 'treat' foods. It is perfectly fine to grate a carrot, zucchini or parsnip into your next batch of baking, but do not make that the only time your tiny human consumes her vegetables. For one thing, do not fool yourself, there is no way she will get enough vegetables (and all their vital nutrients) in her body using this method. And if spinach is pureed into chocolate cake, she is not going to wake up one day and prefer spinach to sweets. She needs to taste both to get an understanding of different flavors and draw her preferences from there.

If vegetables are only connected with (or disguised in) sweet, fluffy, treat foods, this has a danger of creating an unhealthy association that could lead to poor lifestyle choices into adulthood. To ensure healthy food choices are at the forefront, she needs an understanding of why eating vegetables is important, what they really look like and how great they can taste on their own. In other words, all the other ingredients in the 'H-E-A-L-T-H-Y' recipe are necessary.

Lastly, and this may not seem as important, but I like the idea of keeping a treat food as just that. Personally, I want to sit down and enjoy a delicious slice of cake that does not have zucchini hidden in it. I like the idea of a healthy, well-balanced diet that includes the joy of savoring each bite of a rich homemade chocolate brownie or decadent cheesecake once in a while.

RECIPES

Check out the Recipes section for some absolutely fantastic hidden food recipes, including our family favorite spaghetti bolognaise, a basic green smoothie, a vegetable soup made with peanut butter and a great vegetable sauce (in which your child can dip carrots— double vegetable intake!). And yes, there is one zucchini cake recipe included, but please do not make this your go-to for every meal.

There are entire cookbooks dedicated to this concept. The two most popular ones are *Deceptively Delicious* and *The Sneaky Chef*. See the Reference section.

We have now reached the final party of the 'H-E-A-L-T-H-Y' recipe for vegetable success—Yummy Fun. Jump into the next chapter to find some awesome tips for helping your youngsters love vegetables wholeheartedly.

ACTION ITEM

Check out the Recipes section and try a new hidden vegetable recipe this week.

15

HEALTHY INGREDIENT SEVEN (Y) – YUMMY FUN

> 'Approach love and cooking with reckless abandon.' – Dalai Lama

INFUSE WITH HAPPINESS

Eating vegetables does not have to be something your family endures day in and day out, nor hidden away—it should be fun. It needs to be fun. The habit of eating vegetables will not be sustained unless there is some joy attached to it.

Imagine a world where we could get all our nutrients and sustenance from a pill (like that blueberry bubblegum that goes all wrong at Willy Wonka's chocolate factory). Taking a pill would remove all the sensory pleasure we gain from food—the smells, textures and tastes. It would remove all the mental, physical and social aspects of deciding on, preparing and sitting down to a meal. What a dreary, sad world that would be.

What are the best types of Yummy Fun to associate with eating vegetables? How to bring this about without spending a whole lot of time in the hot kitchen? What if an idea you have doesn't work? Answers to these questions and a bazillion great ideas are all in this chapter.

Main 'Yummy Fun' Strategies

There are FIVE main fun vegetables strategies. Yes, five. I could not narrow it down. These are:

- Use rewards and incentives
- Enhance the presentation
- Make them work for it
- Grow a garden
- Play with your food

There are a LOT of great ideas here. Do not try all of them, especially not in the same week. Pick out one or two that you think may work taking into consideration your energy levels, time constraints and your child's personality. Think of it like a fun science experiment. Hypothesize then test. If something works, use the idea again. Most importantly, enjoy the process. This is supposed to be fun.

Use of Rewards and Incentives

Using rewards and incentives can be a fun, low-key way to get your child to start eating vegetables or improve his table manners. Used only for a limited time to motivate certain behavior, it can be very effective way of implementing change with your tiny humans.

Just so we are all on the same page, here are a couple of definitions:

- **Reward** – a benefit provided in recognition of achievement and given afterwards
- **Incentive** – a benefit to motivate an individual to improve his behavior, promised beforehand

In theory at least, internal drivers are much more important than external rewards. There are three keys for keeping motivation high:

- knowing the purpose behind the task
- mastery of the task (a desire to improve)
- autonomy (control over the task)

If anything is a reward in itself, then learning to eat healthy is it. It ticks the purpose, mastery and autonomy aspects in spades. Sometimes these are not enough to drive behavior. So what are your other options?

The most important thing is to find the 'something' that motivates your child to change or improve her behavior. If she doesn't care about the 'something,' then it won't be effective. As discussed earlier, try not to make this something a dessert or a sweet treat or else you are likely to end up in a worse spot than where you started.

If you are worried that you will have to use an external reward to get peas down your child's throat till the end of time, that is also not likely to happen. Rewards tend to have a natural ability to fade in appeal over time and the desired behavior usually sticks.

Behaviors that you may wish to incentivize around vegetables will likely to be along the lines of either:

- eating all (or most of) the vegetables on his plate (make sure it is only a tiny portion to start with)
- trying a bite or tasting a new type of vegetable

The types of incentives and rewards you can use are only limited by your imagination. Remember the important thing is finding out what motivates the tiny human and using that. Here are some suggestions:

- Call Grandma to tell her about trying eggplant for the first time
- Allow some screen time (TV or computer game) after dinner
- Access to a special toy that is kept out of reach most of the time
- A certificate of achievement (easy to make at home)
- A small gift of some stickers, a toy, a book or a wrapped surprise (works well, especially as part of a lunchbox)
- A special outing, perhaps to a restaurant to show off the mastered table manners
- Sticker charts (more below)

Mama Story – The vegetable chart we introduced when he was about four had no reward as such. We drew a picture of any new vegetable tasted on the chart and he would get to color it in. Then he would get to draw smiley faces next to each vegetable he ate at dinner each night. It worked well for him as he loves drawing. He was only eating three vegetables and we expanded it to about 15. I suppose if a kid preferred stickers they would work just as well. We don't use it anymore and he eats all the vegetables just fine. – Alana

Sticker charts can be an excellent form of encouragement. They are easy to implement and inexpensive. Plus, studies have shown that they work in increasing vegetable consumption. Even after the phase of using them has passed, children will still eat more vegetables overall.

Get an old piece of paper and stick it to the wall inside or just outside of your kitchen. Keep it low enough for little hands to be able to place stickers on it. Buy some stickers in advance and keep them out of sight. Dish out the stickers for the behavior you want to encourage.

Sometimes, putting a sticker on the chart is enough of a reward. Alternatively, you can offer a sticker, and then after your child has received say ten of them, you can give her a little present like a book or toy. Some children respond well to the sticker chart. Others do not. If your child eats five beans and then asks for a sticker, then you are onto a winner.

ENHANCE THE PRESENTATION

There are all sorts of easy ways to enhance the presentation of vegetables or the whole meal and thereby increase the likelihood of making the food seem more desirable. These include giving it a flourish, miniaturizing it, cutting it into something familiar or silly or making the whole plate fun.

GIVE IT A FLOURISH

How does your favorite restaurant present a plate to you? Is everything dumped onto a plate and smacked down in front of you? No? Well why not add a bit of flourish with your family. Try one of these ideas:

- On the table—add napkins, some flowers and the 'only kept for special occasion' cutlery and plates.
- On the plate—add a squiggle of sauce (ketchup will do) or some fresh herbs (for instance, a sprinkle of parsley).
- Use ideas from different cultures, such as presenting in a Japanese style 'Bento' box (homemade or bought) with different parts of the meal in different compartments. Children absolutely LOVE this. In absence of an actual Bento box, use a muffin or ice cube tray.

This type of attention to detail often suits a child with a visual learning style, who likes things to be aesthetically pleasing, or gets easily bored with the same old thing. Note that none of these ideas actually ask you to prepare or cook vegetables any differently from how you normally would, they just ask for a bit of presentation pizazz.

MINIATURIZE IT

Everyone likes things that are smaller than they are supposed to be. Think ponies, think high tea sandwiches, think handbag dogs (actually that last one can be a little scary). Find smaller versions of your child's favorite greens or create a smaller version of a vegetable by cutting it up.

- naturally small – cherry tomatoes, baby peas, baby carrots, those tiny corn cob things you find in Chinese takeaways, etc.
- cut up small – one stalk of broccoli, the leaves off the Brussels sprout, strips of pepper, etc.

Mama Tip - Baby spinach leaves (small), baby carrots, baby peas, sugar snap pea pods, cubes of carrot and capsicum and anything really. Broccoli florets, cauliflower florets, sliced mushrooms. Dicing is your friend. No cutting, minimal chewing - LOL! Raw is good. – Annabelle

Most vegetables are easily consumed if lightly steamed or microwaved, but (especially if given raw) keep watching your little ones if you are worried about the risk of choking.

There are added bonuses to this method. The vegetables are often easier to eat as they fit nicely in little hands and mouths. The dish is small enough to not seem overwhelming to your tiny human, so they tend to eat it all. Also, for toddlers and very young children, there is extra practice on their pincer grips between their fingers and thumbs.

FUN OR FAMILIAR

You don't need to just cut the vegetables smaller—you can change up how the food is configured. Vegetables can be cut into many shapes. Use a cookie cutter or a spiralizer. Think long peels of carrot, or cucumbers cut into strips. This would suit a child who is already a bit adventurous.

Alternatively, if your child doesn't like the look of anything new, make the vegetables look like things you know they already like. I started this journey with kale chips—kale baked to crunch like potato chips. Worked a treat with my three-year-old. Other things can be made to look like chips or fries—carrots, parsnips, even beans in a cup. Yes, you don't want to do this for every meal, but it doesn't create a problem if it is done judiciously.

Make the Whole Plate Fun

If you have a bit more time and want to entertain your inner child while getting your actual child to eat more vegetables, then you can go all out and make the whole plate fun.

I hope you read these suggestions and start to feel excited, not exhausted! When she is at college your child is not going to appreciate you turning up with her broccoli tree montage dinner in her dorm room. But your five-year-old will love you for it.

There are entire books dedicated to this (see the Reference Section), but here are a few ideas:

- **Faces** – Use a base of yogurt or soup in a bowl or a piece of bread cut in a circle and add eyes using peas, cut up carrot rounds, cucumbers, radish, etc., plus add a mouth with a strip of any kind of vegetable.
- **Scenes** – What about a broccoli forest on a bed of mashed potato, perhaps with a carrot 'sun'? Or make a rainbow using different colored vegetables —strips of red pepper, grated orange carrot, kernels of yellow corn, etc.
- **Animals** – A lion face with a mane of grated carrots, a caterpillar using cut up cucumbers as the body with a sliced red pepper face and peas for eyes.

Mama Story - My mother-in-law swears she used to put

her eldest daughter's vegetables into mashed potato and serve it to her in an ice-cream cone! – Kayla

MAKE THEM WORK FOR IT

As mentioned in the 'Hide 'Em' chapter, sometimes it is sometimes better to enlist your little one's help to grate the zucchini into the omelet as he is even more likely to eat it than if you sneak the pureed vegetables in by yourself.

Most of the time, when your child has a hand in preparing the meal, she will prefer to eat it. In management speak, active participation enhances engagement in the outcome of the task. Another great reason for putting your child to work is that it connects with her natural curiosity. For instance, if this is mixed with this, then it turns this color. You also trust your child with tasks and give her more independence. Plus, giving her some control over decision making around food means that not only is she likely to eat the vegetables she just helped to choose and prepare, but she also learns to self-assess whether she would like seconds. So it helps her work out her body signals around hunger and fullness.

Other benefits include illustrious outcomes such as the fact that multi-sensory engagement makes learning come alive. It also builds on your relationships as you create a happy team that prepares and cooks together. It can also (but not always) save you time. It can definitely save you from doing the more menial tasks. Many kids actually like the boring, repetitive tasks like washing potatoes, setting the table, stirring and grating. Plus, it allows children to feel like they are doing work and contributing to the household, an important value to hold.

So get your child involved in all parts of meal preparation and reap the benefits at the other end with a child who is keen as a bean to, well, eat beans.

At the Store

This can start at the supermarket or store. There are so many opportunities for getting your tiny human to 'help' you, after a while you may think she is actually helping you. Before you go to the supermarket, ask her what items you are out of, with special care to lead her toward discussing fruit and vegetables. She can watch you make a list, or scribble or draw one as well.

At the store, she will get to see vegetables up close and often in their most natural form. Get her to pick up an avocado and decide if it is ripe or not (hint – the color alone won't tell you, but if you can press the stem bit on the top down, then it's probably perfect to eat). Ask her to count the carrots as you put them in a bag. Invite her to choose a vegetable that she doesn't recognize and then go home and cook it. You may have to Google 'how to cook swede' but so what? Ask her what her favorite vegetable is and allow her to select it herself. See if she can work out what it looks like without guidance.

Mama Story - They come to the vegetable store and look at what's available. If they ask if we can buy it to try, I oblige. If they only try it and don't like it, I still see it as a win. – Deanna

PREPARING AND COOKING

There are so many things your child, even a very young one, can do in the kitchen. Yes it may mean a slower way of doing things, and it may mean more mess, but if it also means more vegetables into little tummies, then it is a win. It is a good idea to invest in a stool or little chair for her to stand on, and perhaps a little apron to wear. Actually, buy the apron anyway—your child will look ultra cute in it.

Involving them in cooking starts with working out what to cook, so why not ask them what they would like for dinner? Give them some recipe options to choose from or show them the pictures in the cookbook that you are prepared to make that week or that night.

She can wash or scrub vegetables. Washing lettuce and then putting it in a salad spinner is a particular favorite. Filling the sink about a quarter full with water and scrubbing a few potatoes is often considered fun as it involves a bit of water, dirt and an opportunity to splash around a bit.

From two years old, kids can pod peas, wash fruit and vegetables, tear up lettuce leaves for the salad and start to try and set the table. From four, kids can slice soft things with a blunt knife, squeeze citrus or mix the salad dressing. When he is a bit older and with a bit more guidance, you can ask him stir the soup or chop the herbs or salad vegetables up. You may be in for a surprise at just how fast your little one learns and how eager he is to help.

Daddy Tip - Decorating pizzas is good for kids too, if they are school age or if you have a lot of patience. – James

GROW A GARDEN

Growing some vegetables is an asset for most families. It would particularly suit children who like learning about how things come about, who are active and love being outside.

First, let's hit some of your objections on the head. No, you don't have to grow a big garden. It's not 1860, and you don't have to feed your family from your land. It is not going to replace all your fruit and vegetable purchases; it won't even come close. At home we have a three-by-six-foot box and some plant pots. You don't even have to have any land at all! You can start with planter boxes or pots on the balcony or even the windowsill. You don't have to maintain a garden all year round. And you don't have to have a green thumb and produce perfect looking vegetables. The fun of gardening is the trial and error and the inherent messiness.

> *Mama Story – The kids have friends over and the amount of kids who we have had around and do not know what some of the vegetables are in our garden shocks me. – Nora*

There are so many benefits to growing your own garden, they could fill a book by themselves. Here is a sample:

- Health benefit 1 – Fresh, organic, seasonal vegetables are not only incredibly tasty, but also have super nutritional value.
- Health benefit 2 – Digging and planting a garden gives you and your child time out in the fresh air

absorbing vitamin D from the sun, and it naturally aids movement and strength.

- Education benefits – Your child learns how vegetables grow in seasons, when best to pick them (the tomatoes must turn red, the beans grow big enough), that vegetables do not have to look perfect to be eaten and what vegetables really look like in their pure natural state. In other words, your kid learns where food actually comes from.
- Planning, patience and the value of work benefits – Children learn when to plant to get the best chance of success, that they have to wait and that a garden takes a bit of work with watering and pulling weeds to ensure the best results.
- Family time benefits – What a cheap, easy and fun way to spend a few minutes a day with your little one. And during the summer he can help water the garden after dinner, thereby saving on having to have a bath (he will get absolutely soaked in the process)!
- Cost benefits – Buy one packet of seeds and with a few parts luck, sunshine and water, you will have cucumbers all summer long.
- Community and social benefits – You are likely to have so many cucumbers that your friends and neighbors get one every time they drop by. What a great small gift to offer loved ones. It costs practically nothing and your child gets to see you as a giving person.

Imagine if everyone had a small garden and grew something different, and during times of surplus you swapped your lovingly grown produce with neighbors and friends. The gift of giving would be enhanced in your community.

I hope I have gotten you incredibly excited about growing a garden and you are ready to start one today. First things first, buy a gardening book or look online for exact details of how and when to plant. This is not such a book.

Why don't you ask your child what he would like to grow? Go to the garden center together and buy some seeds or seedlings of two types of vegetables. Buy a couple of plant pots or set aside a little area in your backyard to add some dirt to. Then plant them.

Favorites with young children include string beans, peas in pods, cherry tomatoes and cucumbers. Also, herbs like parsley and mint are family favorites (see below). You of course can also grow fruit, and strawberries are a fantastic thing to start with. Warning—the food may not make it to the table but instead be eaten by little ones straight from the plant or vine. And that is awesome. Encourage it.

> *Mama Story – The girls love eating straight out of the garden. They will eat a tomato like you would eat apple, carrying it around and crunching into it just the same. I often pick pea pods out of the garden or a bunch of parsley and wash it and leave it on the table. Just as is. The girls often breeze past and graze at it. Before you know it's all gone! It's like vegetable guerrilla warfare - they don't know what's hit them. – Annabelle*

As you get more confident you can get more adventurous. Try growing interesting looking vegetables, or ones that you do not see often at the store. At the moment we have a plant sprouting purple-black peppers. Why not try candy-striped beetroot, purple carrots or kohlrabi (look it up). And two words to encourage really adventurous (and kind of cool) eating—edible flowers. Think zucchini blossoms, pansies, dandelions and violets. If it does not work, the great thing about a garden is you can try something else.

If you have absolutely no room for a garden—perhaps you live in an apartment—why not try to grow some herbs on your windowsill? Parsley is a superfood. Its special powers including protecting our bodies from damaging pollution. Many children absolutely love picking the leaves and eating them straight from the plant. Other herbs that are easy to grow and add a flavor punch to meals include rosemary, thyme, cilantro/coriander, chives and mint.

PLAY WITH YOUR FOOD (YES REALLY)

If you want your child to eat his vegetables, then invite him to play with them. 'Gah. No', you say. 'I have just spent the best part of many previous mealtimes asking him to NOT play with his food. Now you are telling me it is perfectly acceptable?'

Well of course, it is up to you and your tolerance levels on mess and whether you are in a rush to get out the door. However, occasionally it may assist with getting more vegetables into the mouth and hence body of your little one, so it is worth a try.

If you think about it, vegetables practically invite playfulness by their very nature. They have such different looks, textures and colors, it is easy to think of ways to play games with them.

. . .

IMAGINATIVE PLAY

Some ideas do not have to be messy at all—they can just be an exercise in imagination. As part of your 'vegetables are wonderful' conversations, you can ask your child to come up with new names for the vegetables on her plate, the sillier the better. Adding their names to the vegetable can sometimes work too ('Ben's Beans'). Or try to talk health benefits in a surreptitious manner by, for instance, naming them 'X-Ray Vision Carrots'. You could associate vegetables with superheroes, dinosaurs or princesses—'Eat up your Brontosaurus broccoli'.

Mama Story - It also helps if he knows one of his heroes eats it like Fireman Sam eats spinach. – Olivia

Daddy Tip – I tell the kids that they are giraffes so they need to eat the 'trees' (broccoli) with their long tongues. – Rob

Older kids can be presented with a few different colored vegetables and be invited to imagine the 'painting' what will happen in their tummies when they eat them. The orange carrot sun, the broccoli trees, the other bright colors from spinach, tomato or beets. They will surprise you with how imaginative they can be. There will be whole landscapes down the hatch and described after each mouthful.

HANDS-ON PLAY

For the more sensory child who exhibits more practical tendencies or learns in a kinesthetic way, then getting down and dirty may be the key to ingesting more vegetables.

See if your child wants to eat with his hands. Younger children find it easier to eat something when they don't have to use a fork. This becomes even more inviting (and more messy) when there is a dip or a sauce in which to dunk raw cut up vegetables. Try natural yogurt, sour cream, hummus, ketchup or a vegetable dip (see Recipes chapter).

Being more hands-on doesn't have to end with cut up, raw vegetables. Mashed potato can be 'finger painted' and corn on the cob practically begs for a hands-on experience. Vegetable soup can be presented in a cup to drink (make sure it's not too hot), or slurped at the end of the bowl. Yes it may be considered a bit rude, but think of all those vegetable nutrients in the soup water being ingested.

Mama Tip - Kids always love tacos or build-a-burger, that way they can at least choose which vegetables they like without any fuss. – Raquel

Parents may despair, especially if looks like more is going on the floor than into little mouths, but it is all learning and familiarization, and the more familiar we are with things the more likely we are to want to try them and embrace eating them.

If you really want to encourage a bit of fun but without the mess, you can aid the eating in a playful manner. Many toddlers embrace a bit of 'airplane' or 'choo-choo train' action to get whatever is on the spoon into their mouths. Or the green bean could turn into a jumping bean and you could bounce it all the way to your young child —boing, boing, boing, crunch! They could say 'hello' to the pea on the plate and then 'goodbye' as it disappears down their throats. This may be slightly more labor intensive up front but less messy afterwards.

FUN FOR THE WHOLE FAMILY

A few times a year you could switch it up a bit and get into a whole day of food-related fun. This involves a bit of planning and is best saved for the holidays or a lazy weekend. Creating traditions and lasting positive memories is not only good for health in a nutritional sense but also in mental and social context as well.

When they grow up, your children won't remember the breakfast you made for them each morning, but they will remember 'Backwards Day'.

What Is 'Backwards Day'? It is a day when you eat your meals back to front. You have dinner for breakfast and breakfast for dinner (lunch can take care of itself). Kids find this hilarious. And you can get them to eat vegetables at breakfast time. Yes you heard it right. **Vegetables at breakfast**. Breakfast on this day could be a Mediterranean buffet style breakfast that includes cut up feta cheese, tomatoes and cucumber with hummus and other dips and fresh bread or crackers. Or you can switch it up completely and eat spaghetti or barbecue or fried rice (all with some vegetables thrown into the meal).

Dinner can be scrambled eggs or an omelet with some spinach thrown in, or pancakes with a selection of fruit. That last option did not have vegetables, but remember, your family ALREADY HAD VEGETABLES AT BREAKFAST!

Another popular day is 'Pirate Day'. Pirate Day is best sprung on the kid when you arrive in her room with an eye patch on and a toy parrot on your shoulder announcing it is 'Annual Pirate Day'. Have costumes for everyone at the ready. It is mandatory to spend all day talking like a pirate (say 'Arrrr', and 'Ahoy Me Maties' at every opportunity). Food associated with Pirate Day is completely at your discretion. Check out the Pinterest boards for inspiration. Maybe organize a treasure hunt that leads to a picnic, or serve up fish or stew. Just leave the rum for the grown-ups.

If a whole day of fun is not within the realm of possibility, then why not change up the location of dinner once in a while? Have dinner on the living room floor (with a large cloth put down) or outside in the backyard.

> *Mama Tip – For a change, I will also let them eat on the trampoline or on a rug on the deck. Making tea fun. – Nora*

I hope these ideas have piqued your imagination and you are already working out a good time to schedule in Pirate Day or Backwards Day.

ASSOCIATIONS

One of my fondest memories from when I was a little girl was eating beans straight off the vine in my grandparents' vegetable patch. I have such nostalgia about this that beans were one of the first vegetables we planted in our own garden.

There are plenty of ideas in this big chapter. You may realize by now that it does not matter what you choose to start with. What is important is the associations that are made.

Vegetables can indeed be a tasty treat. Growing, cooking and making meals with vegetables can be fun and enjoyable. Eating them is not just something you do out of habit, but can be a welcome pleasure. The more you and your family associate happiness with vegetables, the more likely your kids will effortlessly choose them, and therefore remain healthy throughout their childhoods and into their adult lives.

People keep up habits that they enjoy. Yes it is critical to make eating vegetables a normal, everyday habit, but without this core component, fun, it is unlikely that the habit will be maintained.

Don't just create habits, create rituals. Do something that ends up becoming a fond memory for your own kids, a recollection that just happens to include salad.

The next chapter has a few final thoughts on healthy eating, parenting and life. The last two chapters contain a handy quick reference summary and some easy and delicious recipes.

ACTION ITEM

Pick one 'Yummy Fun' idea and introduce it as soon as you can.

16

FINAL THOUGHTS

> 'It is easier to change a man's religion than to change his diet.' - Margaret Mead

THIS BOOK IS ABOUT ENCOURAGING YOUR CHILD TO EAT MORE vegetables, but deep down it is about YOU. On the journey from picky to adventurous, from unhealthy to wellness, I have no doubt that you will discover even more about yourself as a parent, a teacher and a human being.

What you are trying to ingrain into your children's identities is that they love eating vegetables, that they like being healthy and embracing new things. This may be something that you are attempting to carve out for yourself as well if you have lost it over the years.

There is a saying that you write the book that you need to read yourself. I have no doubt that has been the case here. But what surprised me the most was how ingrained some of my unhealthy beliefs were. I could gather together all the tips and tricks in the universe, but if I still believed that my children should 'finish their plates', or that I could not stand the waste or messy fun, or I disliked the feeling of rejection so much I didn't have the motivation to try something new, then nothing would really change.

Just like everyone has the right to choose what they put in their mouths, you also have the right to decide what you put in your head. Changing your mindset is the key to success.

At the end of the day, providing healthy food for your family is all about LOVE. At times, you may feel mean, but by being fed nutritious meals in a secure environment, your children feel valued and this allows them to naturally make healthier choices. It is not 'tough love'—it is just love.

So lift your head out of this book, take a deep breath, and smile. Go and find the tiny human and give her an enormous hug. Overload him with smoochy kisses. Tell those beautiful children of yours that you love them to the moon and back and always will.

17

BUSY PARENT SUMMARY

SHOW ME THE MONEY

Okay, how many of you skipped straight here? Tut tut. What naughty busy parents you are. However, in this age of short attention spans and insane busyness, it is to be expected.

Whether you leapt straight here or took the time to really understand the reasoning and benefits behind each of the strategies, this summary gives you all the good stuff without the fluff.

VEGETABLE EATING GOALS FOR THE WHOLE FAMILY

- As part of '5+ A Day' it is recommended to have three portions (handfuls) of vegetables as an absolute minimum per day.
- Three portions equates to about one cup of vegetables for kids under five years old and two cups for over fives.

- Most people can safely and beneficially DOUBLE the amount of vegetables in their diet.
- This equates to six to eight handfuls or two to four cups of vegetables over the course of the day.
- Another way to view this goal is to aim for non-starchy vegetables taking up half the plate at lunch and dinner.

H-E-A-L-T-H-Y Ingredients and Strategies

Seven ingredients make up a 'H-E-A-L-T-H-Y' recipe to encourage your children to eat and love vegetables and promote healthy eating in your family. Each of the ingredients has a handful of strategies that you can pick and implement to move from fussy to healthy.

Habit – create habits around eating vegetables

Encourage Variety – get a wide variety of vegetables into your kids

Accept and Allow – allow your children to understand their own bodies

Lay Down the Law – add some structure and routine around mealtimes

Talk – communicate with your kids

Hide 'Em– hide vegetables in meals and snacks

Yummy Fun – inject some FUN back into the kitchen

Habit Strategies

There are three main strategies that really work for getting the kids to have an ingrained belief that vegetables are a normal part of daily life. These are:

- Always there—have vegetables and fruit readily available.
- Lead with vegetables—serve a small amount of vegetables before 'the main course' at lunch and dinner.
- Vegetables at every meal—including snacks and even breakfast sometimes.

Tasty tips to get you started with 'Habit' strategies:

- Keep washed, cut up vegetables at eye level in the fridge.
- Try the *'Sacrificial Vegetable'* tactic of placing tiny portions of three different vegetables on a plate, one of which is less favored. Then watch your child happily eat the other two vegetables.
- Get your kids' buy in for vegetables with dinner by giving them a 'choice' between two different types of vegetables or ways of cooking them.

Encourage Variety Strategies

There are three main strategies that help children to become more adventurous eaters. These are:

- Exposure—introduce a tiny portion of a vegetable up to 20 times.
- Embrace the inherent variety in vegetables—color, texture, taste, etc.

- Present vegetables in different ways or in different settings.

Tasty tips to get you started on with 'Variety' strategies:

- Associate the new vegetable with something your child already finds familiar or likes (peas are 'green corn').
- Try different vegetables in season—they are fresher, tastier and often cheaper.
- Encouraging your child to do other things that are different, (e.g.: listening to different music or trying a different sport) may make them more inclined to try a new food.

ACCEPT AND ALLOW STRATEGIES

There are three main strategies that allow our tiny humans control over their own bodies. These are:

- Follow Satter's 'Division of Responsibility' (see tips below)
- Reframe hunger—hunger and fullness are not good or bad, but simply different states the body can be in.
- Six magical little words: 'You don't have to eat it.'

Tasty tips to get you started on with 'Accept and Allow' strategies:

- The parent is responsible for what, when, where (of feeding).

- The child is responsible for how much and whether (of eating).
- Sometimes when your children say they are hungry, they may instead be thirsty and actually need a glass of water.

Lay Down the Law Strategies

There are three main strategies to create a structured and secure eating environment in the home. These are:

- A regular mealtime routine—five meals per day with some times when there is no eating allowed.
- Behavior expectations and rules—decide on what table manners are important to you and your family.
- Family mealtimes together—try for at least one meal all together each week (more is better).

Tasty tips to get you started on with 'Lay Down the Law' strategies:

- Have family rules in place for requests for food between mealtimes, especially after dinner (and especially if not much of the meal was eaten).
- Never EVER link getting dessert with finishing all their vegetables.
- Within the rules and structure you have set, try to say 'YES' to your kids as much as possible.

Talk Strategies

There are three main communication strategies that improve the chances of your kids embracing the whole eating vegetables paradigm shift. These are:

- Praise and encouragement—show your love to your child.
- Embrace the inherent greatness of vegetables—talk them up!
- Model the behavior that you want—show your love of vegetables.

Tasty tips to get you started on with 'Talk' strategies:

- Let your kids know that *The Guinness Book of Records* lists avocado as the most nutritionally complete fruit in the world.
- Try 'Color Week' when each family dinner meal is one color, e.g.: 'Monday Green Night', 'Tuesday Red Night', etc.
- Allow your kids to try something off your plate that they normally would not eat as a kind of treat or privilege, e.g.: olives, sun-dried tomato.

HIDE 'EM STRATEGIES

There are three main hide vegetables strategies. These are:

- Hide vegetables in 'normal' dishes like pasta, soup, curry, pie, etc.
- Hide vegetables in plain sight on pizza, in sushi, wrapped, etc.
- Hide vegetables in cakes and treat foods (WARNING!)

Tasty tips to get you started on with 'Hide 'Em' strategies:

- See how many vegetables you can cram into one dish. Can you beat six in the spaghetti bolognaise recipe below?
- Encourage your child to 'help' you hide vegetables e.g.: grate the zucchini that is mixed with the scrambled eggs.
- Hide some finely diced peppers or peas in your child's penne then invite them to 'treasure hunt' for the vegetables, a game many little kids love.

YUMMY FUN STRATEGIES

There are FIVE main strategies to inject some fun around preparing, cooking and eating vegetables. These are:

- Use rewards and incentives.
- Enhance the presentation—give it a flourish, miniaturize it, cut it into shapes or make the whole plate look fun (like a face or animal).
- Make them work for it—shopping, preparing, cooking.
- Grow a garden.
- Play with your food—imaginative play, hands-on play, fun for the whole family.

Tasty tips to get you started on with 'Yummy Fun' strategies:

- Present the meal in a Japanese style 'Bento' box (or muffin or ice cube tray) with different parts of the meal in different compartments.

- Getting kids to help in the kitchen makes them feel valued, is likely to up the vegetable intake as they are involved in the preparation AND delegates the boring, repetitive tasks to your little ones—win, win, win!
- Grow a small vegetable garden and watch your kids pick and eat vegetables straight from the garden like "vegetable guerrilla warfare - they don't know what hit them".

ACTION ITEMS

- Present a small platter of vegetables as an appetizer before the main course of dinner tonight.
- Buy a new vegetable that you have not eaten before and get the whole family involved in trying it.
- Practice saying in a calm manner with a smile on your face: "You don't have to eat it".
- Set a date for at least one family dinner this week.
- Heap an extraordinary amount of praise onto your child for some desired behavior at dinner tonight (however small) and notice the response.
- Try a new hidden vegetable recipe this week – see Recipes.
- Pick one 'Yummy Fun' idea and introduce it as soon as you can e.g.: make the plate look fun to eat, cook together, grow a vegetable garden or plan 'Backwards Day'.

18

RECIPES

What We Want

As parents we want meals eaten without fussing, without whining and certainly without outright rejection. We want to create quick, simple, tasty and nutritious meals the whole family will love.

We want a mealtime guarantee!

All these meals and snacks below have been created and tested by busy parents just like you with great levels of success. Maybe not every meal will suit every child, but you are guaranteed to find at least one family favorite in this list.

Note that the lunch and dinner recipes are meant for a family of two adults and two or three children.

BREAKFAST

· · ·

Green Breakfast Smoothie for One (or Maybe Two Tiny Humans)

Ingredients

1 chopped frozen banana

Handful frozen berries (any type)

Large handful spinach leaves

Approximately 1 cup water or coconut water

-

Remove any large stalks from spinach and finely chop.

Put all ingredients into a blender until smooth.

Add more water if required.

Tip – This can be put into ice cube trays and frozen into ice blocks for a hot summer's day—a real treat!

Vegetable Omelet for One (or Maybe Two Tiny Humans)

Ingredients

2 eggs

Salt and pepper

Fresh herbs like parsley, chives, basil

Your choice of vegetable(s): spinach, tomato, pepper, mushroom, onion, peas

Handful of grated cheese (optional)

Butter or oil (optional)

Break eggs into a bowl, whisk lightly and add salt and pepper.

Pour into a hot pan (sizzling with a little butter or oil).

Scatter in a teaspoon or two of herbs.

Then add a tablespoon or two of finely diced raw vegetable(s)—if it is spinach, then lightly sauté it first.

Add grated cheese if desired.

Once egg has set on the bottom (2 or 3 minutes), use a spatula to fold the sides in like a parcel, then turn over and cook for a couple more minutes.

Remove and serve, with or without toast.

Savory Cheese Muffins

Ingredients

2 cups flour (standard or half whole wheat)

1 tsp baking powder

½ tsp baking soda

Salt and pepper (optional)

2 eggs

1 cup milk

¼ cup butter, melted

1 bunch scallion/spring onion

1 pepper

½ cup grated cheese

-

Preheat oven to 400°F (200 C)

Coat a 12-hole muffin tray with cooking spray or use cupcake paper.

Combine flour, baking powder, baking soda, pepper and salt in a large bowl.

Whisk eggs, milk and melted butter in a medium bowl.

Finely dice scallions and pepper and fold in about half a cup each into wet mixture.

Add grated cheese to wet mixture and mix all together.

Make a well in the center of the dry ingredients and add the wet ingredients and mix until just combined.

Scoop the mixture into the muffin tray (so the cups are about 2/3 full).

Bake the muffins until the tops are golden brown about 20 minutes.

Cool in the tray for 5 minutes and then turn the muffins out onto a wire rack to cool slightly before serving.

Makes 12 muffins for a few days' worth of breakfasts on the go.

LUNCH

VEGETABLE SOUP WITH PEANUT BUTTER

The peanut butter may sound like a strange addition, but try it and be amazed!

Ingredients

1 onion

½ leek

3 large carrots

1 large parsnip

1 large potato

¼ pumpkin (optional)

1 large bunch of spinach, washed

4 or 5 cups of reduced or no salt vegetable stock (bought or homemade)

4 tbsp of smooth peanut butter

-

Peel and roughly chop carrots, parsnip, potato and pumpkin.

Place onion and garlic in a large pot and gently fry for a few minutes.

Place all the vegetables apart from the spinach in the pot, cook for a few minutes then cover with the stock.

Bring to the boil and then reduce heat to a simmer.

Cook for approximately 40 minutes or until vegetables are very soft and starting to break up.

Add the spinach and cook for another 5 minutes.

Remove from the heat and add the peanut butter.

Use a stick blender and blend until nearly smooth.

Add a dollop of natural yogurt or sour cream and a sprinkle of freshly chopped parsley to serve.

FRITTERS/CORN FRITTERS

Ingredients

1 cup flour

1 standard can of creamed corn (400g/14 oz.)

1 large or 2 small eggs

1 tsp salt

1 tbsp freshly chopped parsley

2 tsp sweet chili sauce (remove if you children do not like it spicy)

Choose two or three finely diced or grated vegetables, e.g.: ½ pepper (any color), ½ carrot, ½ zucchini, ½ cup frozen baby peas, 1 cup of spinach or chard (silverbeet), etc.

-

Pour creamed corn into a bowl and add salt, egg, sweet chili sauce, parsley and any vegetables of your choice.

Mix well, then add flour and mix again.

Heat a little oil in a frying pan and drop a few spoonfuls of mixture into pan.

Cook on each side about 3 minutes, until brown.

Serve with hummus or homemade tomato or vegetable sauce and a small salad.

Makes 5 to 10 depending on size of fritter.

Tip - For lighter and fluffier fritters, separate the egg(s) and whisk the egg white separately until stiff and add at the end of the mix.

Rice Paper Rolls (that the kids can make)

Ingredients

1 packet (about 8 to 10 sheets) rice paper

2 cups of glass noodles

1 scallion or spring onion

1 cup lettuce leaves

1 carrot

½ cucumber

Handful bean sprouts (if available)

2 tbsp cilantro or coriander (optional)

2 tbsp mint (optional)

1 lemon or lime

1 tsp sweet chili sauce

-

Soak noodles in warm water for 15 minutes until softened, then drain.

Finely slice scallion, carrot, cucumber and (optional) herbs and shred lettuce into small pieces.

Place noodles in bowl with all vegetables.

Add the juice of lemon and sweet chili sauce and mix all to combine.

Dip each sheet of rice paper briefly into warm water to wet it (but don't soak it) and lay on a flat surface.

Spoon about ¼ to 1/3 cup of noodle mixture onto center of rice paper.

Fold in ends of rice paper and roll up tightly (slice up if required).

Chill until ready to serve or demolish immediately with a dipping sauce of your choice.

DINNER

MR. S's SPAGHETTI BOLOGNAISE

Ingredients

250g premium mince/10 oz. ground beef

1 onion

1 carrot

1 celery stalk

½ to 1 pepper (any color)

½ to 1 zucchini

2 cups or large handfuls of spinach or chard (silverbeet), stalks optional

1 standard can of plain chopped tomatoes in juice (400g/14 oz.)

½ cup tomato paste (or pasta sauce)

Finely chopped fresh herbs—parsley, chives, thyme, rosemary, or use dried

¼ tsp Vegemite (optional and only if it is available where you live)

250g/10 oz. uncooked pasta or spaghetti—any type

1 cup grated cheese (optional)

-

Finely chop or dice all vegetables and grate carrot if preferred.

Fry onion in large pan with a little olive oil until color changes, approx. 3 minutes.

Add grated carrot to pan and cook for a further few minutes (optional: put lid on to cook faster).

Add meat (and optional Vegemite) and break up so it cooks faster.

Once meat is brown add all other chopped vegetables and cook for a while until soft.

Add can of tomatoes and tomato paste (or sauce).

Mix all ingredients together and turn down the heat to medium-low to simmer for 10 to 15 minutes.

Boil pasta in saucepan of boiling water until al dente (approx. 10-15 minutes) then drain.

Serve a portion of pasta and the meat and vegetables mix in a bowl and sprinkle some cheese on top.

NOTE: If you do not have some of the vegetables in the list above, substitute for what you do have or leave out completely.

• • •

BUILD A BURGER

Ingredients

250g premium mince / 10 oz. ground beef

1 egg

1 onion

1 carrot

1 zucchini

1 cup spinach or chard (silverbeet)—stalks removed

Handful fresh herbs like parsley

¼ to ½ cup of breadcrumbs and/or rolled oats

Salt and pepper

Burger buns or pita breads

Selection of burger fillings: lettuce, tomato, cheese, gherkins, pineapple, beetroot, fried egg, fried onion

Selection of burger sauces: ketchup, BBQ, mayonnaise, satay, aioli or any other family favorite

-

Finely dice onion, peel and grate carrot and zucchini and chop spinach/chard.

Finely dice herbs.

Put meat, egg, vegetables, herbs and breadcrumbs/rolled oats in a bowl and mix together thoroughly until combined.

With wet hands roll mixture into balls and then flatten into burger-sized patties.

Fry patties in a hot pan with a little oil on both sides until completely cooked (brown).

Lightly toast burger buns or pita breads.

Put out a selection of fillings and sauces and invite the family to build a burger.

FRIED RICE

Ingredients

2 cups of uncooked rice—basmati, white or brown are the best options

2 eggs

Your choice of vegetable—have two or three: onion, pepper, mushroom, corn pieces, peas

Soy sauce

Salt and pepper

Cashew nuts (optional)

-

Boil rice or cook in a rice cooker.

Whisk eggs in a small bowl and cook in a small frying pan, set aside.

Finely dice vegetables.

Add all vegetables, including frozen peas, to a large pan and fry with a little oil for a few minutes.

Cut up cooked egg and add to large pan.

Scoop out cooked rice, add to large pan and mix with other ingredients.

Add soy sauce, salt and pepper and cashew nuts to taste, mix through and cook for a few more minutes.

LUNCH OR DINNER (JUST THE VEGETABLE PART)

KALE CHIPS

Ingredients

Bunch of fresh kale

Extra virgin olive oil

Salt and pepper

-

Preheat the oven to about 160 to 170 Celsius (320 F).

Remove the stems from the leaves of three large stalks of kale.

Discard stems, wash and tear leaves.

Line a large oven tray with baking paper and spread kale leaves on it.

Spray or lightly pour olive oil on the leaves, plus season with salt and pepper.

Bake in cool oven until crispy and dried (no longer than 10 minutes).

Tip – Baking kale chips is a fine art—you want them light and crispy, not soggy and not charcoal. This may take more than one batch before you get it just right in your oven.

. . .

GOURMET BROCCOLI

Ingredients

1 small head of broccoli, cut into pieces

Handful of grated cheese

Mixed herbs (fresh or dried)

Red wine

Salt and pepper

-

Lightly steam or microwave broccoli.

Put onto plates or in a serving bowl.

Add grated cheese, a sprinkle of mixed herbs and a couple of drops of red wine plus salt and pepper.

RED COLESLAW

Your little one hates greens? Well not to worry, this is ALL red and orange!

Ingredients - Slaw

½ red cabbage

½ red onion

2 radishes

1 large red pepper

1 large carrot

¼ cup parsley (optional as makes it a bit green)

Ingredients - Dressing

¼ cup olive oil

¼ cup orange juice

2 tablespoons honey

Vinegar or mustard to taste (if the kids like it)

-

Finely slice all the vegetables and toss to combine.

Pour all dressing ingredients into a jar, put a tight lid on and shake.

Add the dressing to the red slaw.

DIPS AND SAUCES

SALLY'S HOMEMADE KETCHUP (TOMATO SAUCE)

Ingredients

2 standard cans of plain chopped tomatoes in juice (400g / 14 oz.)

½ onion, chopped

¼ cup apple cider vinegar

1 tablespoon sugar (optional)

1 teaspoon ground allspice

1 teaspoon ground cinnamon

Salt and pepper

-

Bring all the ingredients to a boil in the saucepan, stirring to dissolve the spices.

Reduce the heat and simmer for about 50 minutes until the sauce reduces by almost half and is quite thick.

Blend with a stick blender or in a food processor.

Store in a clean glass jar in the fridge for up to 1 month.

Tip - If you want to convert this into a spicier BBQ sauce, then add 1 teaspoon Tabasco sauce, 1 tablespoon paprika and 1 tablespoon chili powder to the mix.

VEGETABLE DIP OR SAUCE

Ingredients

1 onion

1 leek, white part only

1 red pepper

1 carrot

1 zucchini

1 standard can of plain chopped tomatoes in juice (400g / 14 oz.)

300ml / 10 oz. (or maybe more) of low or no salt vegetable stock, bought or homemade

Extra virgin olive oil

Salt and pepper

-

Finely dice onion, leek and pepper.

Grate carrot and zucchini.

Cook onion and leek in a covered saucepan on a low heat with a little oil until soft, about 10 minutes.

Add the pepper, carrot and zucchini and cook for a further 3 minutes.

Pour in the can of tomatoes and stock and cook for 20 minutes or until all vegetables are tender.

Use a stick blender and blend until nearly smooth.

Pour into a dish and serve warm or cold with potato wedges or vegetable sticks.

GUACAMOLE

This is a family favorite the kids can make on their own

Ingredients

1 or 2 ripe avocados

1 lemon or lime

¼ tsp cumin

1 clove of garlic (optional)

Dash of Tabasco sauce or ¼ tsp chili powder (optional)

Salt and pepper

-

Cut avocado in half, remove the stone and scoop out all the flesh into a bowl.

Mash the avocado with a fork.

Add the rest of the ingredients and mix together.

Chill until ready or serve immediately with plain corn chips or carrot sticks.

DESSERT OR SWEET SNACK

ZUCCHINI CAKE

Ingredients

3 eggs

1 cup olive oil

1 cup sugar

3 cups of flour

3 tsp cinnamon

1 tsp baking soda

½ tsp baking powder

Pinch of salt

2 tsp vanilla extract

2 zucchini peeled and grated

-

Preheat oven to 180 Celsius (350 F).

Grease a round cake tin or two small loaf tins.

Whisk the eggs, oil and sugar together in a bowl.

Put the dry ingredients (flour, cinnamon, baking soda, baking powder, salt) in a separate large bowl and mix to combine.

To the dry ingredients fold in the egg mix, zucchini and vanilla extract.

Pour into cake tin or loaf tins and bake for about 1 hour.

Take out of the oven, turn onto a wire rack once cooled a little.

Great served warm with a dollop of plain unsweetened yogurt.

READER GIFT: THE HAPPY20

For all you wonderful, busy parents, I created

THE HAPPY20
20 Free Ways to Boost Happiness in 20 Seconds or Less

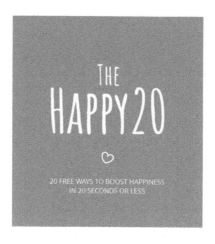

A PDF gift for you with quick ideas to improve mood and add a little sparkle to your day.

Head to **JulieSchooler.com/gift** and grab your copy today.

ABOUT THE AUTHOR

Julie had aspirations of being a writer since she was very young but somehow got sidetracked into the corporate world. After the birth of her first child, she rediscovered her creative side. You can find her at JulieSchooler.com.

Her *Easy Peasy* books provide simple and straightforward information on parenting topics. The *Nourish Your Soul* series shares delicious wisdom to feel calmer, happier and more fulfilled.

Busy people can avoid wasting time searching for often confusing and conflicting advice and instead spend time with the beautiful tiny humans in their lives and do what makes their hearts sing.

Julie lives with her family in a small, magnificent country at the bottom of the world where you may find her trying to bake the perfect chocolate brownie.

facebook.com/JulieSchoolerAuthor
instagram.com/julie.schooler
twitter.com/JulieSchooler

BOOKS BY JULIE SCHOOLER

Easy Peasy **Books**

Easy Peasy Potty Training

Easy Peasy Healthy Eating

Nourish Your Soul Books

Rediscover Your Sparkle

Crappy to Happy

Embrace Your Awesomeness

Bucket List Blueprint

Super Sexy Goal Setting

Find Your Purpose in 15 Minutes

Clutter-Free Forever

Children's Picture Books

Maxy-Moo Flies to the Moon

Collections

Change Your Life 3-in-1 Collection

Rebelliously Happy 3-in-1 Collection

JulieSchooler.com/books

ACKNOWLEDGMENTS

Without a doubt I would not have written this book without the amazing support and accountability provided by a hard-working and creative online community of writers and authors. Thanks again in particular to Stephanie and Marcy.

I have massive appreciation for the busy parents who completed the healthy eating survey. Thank you for taking your time to supply your sometimes horrifying, sometimes hilarious and always straight-up honest answers to the survey questions.

To Andrew and our two beautiful tiny humans, Dylan and Eloise. I live in a perpetual state of astonishment about how fortunate my life is. Thank you for making me laugh every single day.

PLEASE LEAVE A REVIEW

Easy Peasy Healthy Eating

The Busy Parents' Guide to Helping Picky Eaters Love Vegetables

THANK YOU FOR READING THIS BOOK

I devoted many months to researching and writing this book. I then spent more time having it professionally edited, working with a designer to create an awesome cover and launching it into the world.

Time, money and heart has gone into this book and I very much hope you enjoyed reading it as much as I loved creating it.

It would mean the world to me if you could spend a few minutes writing a review on Goodreads or the online store where you purchased this book.

A review can be as short or long as you like and should be helpful and honest to assist other potential buyers of the book.

Reviews provide social proof that people like and recommend the book. More book reviews mean more book sales which means I can write more books.

Your book review helps me, as an independent author, more than you could ever know. I read every single review and when I get five-star review it absolutely makes my day.

Thanks, Julie.

REFERENCES

Websites

5+ A Day www.5aday.co.nz

Claire Turnball www.claireturnbull.co.nz

Choose My Plate www.choosemyplate.gov

Dr. Libby Weaver www.drlibby.com

Ellyn Satter www.ellynsatterinstitute.org

Mindless Eating www.mindlesseating.org

WHO www.who.int

'Six Words' article: www.scarymommy.com/six words that will end picky eating

Books

Accidentally Overweight – Solve Your Weight Loss Puzzle – Dr. Libby Weaver (NZ, 2010)

Beauty from the Inside Out – Enhance the Gifts Nature So Graciously Gave You – Dr. Libby Weaver (NZ, 2013)

Deceptively Delicious – Simple Secrets to Get Your Kids Eating Good Food – Jessica Seinfeld (USA, 2007)

Feel Good for Life – A Recipe for Great Health and Vitality – Claire Turnball (NZ, 2015)

Fighting Globesity – A Practical Guide to Personal Health and Global Sustainability – Phillip and Jackie Mills (NZ, 2007)

French Children Don't Throw Food – Parenting Secrets from Paris - Pamela Druckerman (USA, 2013)

Fun Food for Fussy Little Eaters – How to Get Your Kids to Eat Fruit and Veg – Smita Srivastava (UK, 2013)

Getting to YUM – The 7 Secrets of Raising Eager Eaters – Karen Le Billon (USA, 2014)

Get Your Family Eating Right! – A 30-Day Plan for Teaching Your Kids Healthy Eating Habits for Life - Lynn Fredericks and Mercedes Sanchez (USA, 2013)

Grow Me Well – Nutritional Know-How for Every Body – Dee and Tamarin Pigneguy (NZ, 2013)

Happy Mealtimes for Kids – A Guide to Healthy Eating with Simple Recipes that Children Love – Cathy Glass (UK, 2012)

Healthy Eating for Kids – Over 100 Meal Ideas, Recipes and Healthy Eating Tips for Children – Anita Bean (UK, 2007)

Home for Dinner – Mixing Food, Fun and Conversation for a Happier Family and Healthier Kids – Anne K. Fishel (USA, 2015)

It's Not About the Broccoli – Three Habits to Teach Your Kids for a Lifetime of Healthy Eating – Dina Rose (USA, 2014)

Politically Incorrect Parenting – Before Your Kids Drive You Crazy – Nigel Latta (NZ, 2010)

Raising a Healthy, Happy Eater – A Stage by Stage Guide to Setting Your Child on the Path to Adventurous Eating – N. Fernando and M. Potock (USA, 2015)

River Cottage Baby and Toddler Cookbook – Nikki Duffy (UK, 2011)

Spiralize It! – Creative Spiralizer Recipes for Every Type of Eater – Kenzie Swanhart (USA, 2015)

Stress Free Feeding – How to Develop Healthy Eating Habits in Your Child – Lucy Cooke and Laura Webber (UK, 2015)

The No-Cry Picky Eater Solution – Gentle Ways to Encourage Your Child to Eat – and Eat Healthy – Elizabeth Pantley (USA, 2012)

The Speedy Sneaky Chef – Quick, Healthy Fixes for Your Family's Favorite Packaged Foods – Missy Chase Lapine (USA, 2012)

The Toddler Cafe – Fast, Healthy and Fun Ways to Feed even the Pickiest Eater – Jennifer Carden (US, 2008)

Toddler Taming – The Guide to Your Child from One to Four – Dr. Christopher Green (AUS-NZ, 2001) – Two chapters only

Wild Eats and Adorable Treats – 40 Animal Inspired Meals and Snacks for Kids – Jill Mills (USA, 2015)

Made in the USA
Las Vegas, NV
03 January 2022

39958116R00098